Third Edition

Weight Training

STEPS TO SUCCESS

Thomas R. Baechle, EdD, CSCS,*D; NSCA-CPT,*D

Roger W. Earle, MA, CSCS,*D; NSCA-CPT,*D

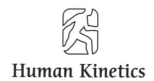

Human Kinetics

Library of Congress Cataloging-in-Publication Data

Baechle, Thomas R., 1943-
    Weight training : steps to success / Thomas R. Baechle, Roger W. Earle.-- 3rd ed.
        p. cm.
    Includes bibliographical references.
    ISBN 0-7360-5533-9 (soft cover)
  1. Weight training.   2. Physical fitness.   I. Earle, Roger W., 1967- II.
Title.
    GV546.B344 2006
    613.7'13--dc22

                                                2005022589

ISBN: 0-7360-5533-9

The Web addresses cited in this text were current as of November, 2005 unless otherwise noted.

Acquisitions Editor: Jana Hunter; **Developmental Editor:** Cynthia McEntire; **Assistant Editor:** Scott Hawkins; **Copyeditor:** Cheryl Ossola; **Proofreader:** Kim Thoren; **Permission Manager:** Carly Breeding; **Graphic Designer:** Nancy Rasmus; **Graphic Artist:** Tara Welsch; **Cover Designer:** Keith Blomberg; **Photographer (cover):** Dan Wendt; **Art Manager:** Kareema McLendon; **Illustrator:** Roberto Sabas; **Printer:** United Graphics

Human Kinetics books are available at special discounts for bulk purchase. Special editions or book excerpts can also be created to specification. For details, contact the Special Sales Manager at Human Kinetics.

Printed in the United States of America   10   9   8   7   6   5   4   3   2   1

Human Kinetics
Web site: www.HumanKinetics.com

United States: Human Kinetics
P.O. Box 5076
Champaign, IL 61825-5076
800-747-4457
e-mail: humank@hkusa.com

Canada: Human Kinetics
475 Devonshire Road Unit 100
Windsor, ON N8Y 2L5
800-465-7301 (in Canada only)
e-mail: orders@hkcanada.com

Europe: Human Kinetics
107 Bradford Road
Stanningley
Leeds LS28 6AT, United Kingdom
+44 (0) 113 255 5665
e-mail: hk@hkeurope.com

Australia: Human Kinetics
57A Price Avenue
Lower Mitcham, South Australia 5062
08 8277 1555
e-mail: liaw@hkaustralia.com

New Zealand: Human Kinetics
Division of Sports Distributors NZ Ltd.
P.O. Box 300 226 Albany
North Shore City
Auckland
0064 9 448 1207
e-mail: info@humankinetics.co.nz

Third Edition

Weight Training

STEPS TO SUCCESS

◪ Contents

☐ Climbing the Steps to Weight Training Success

Get ready to climb a staircase—one that will lead you to become stronger, more fit, and more knowledgeable about weight training. You cannot leap to the top, but you can reach it by climbing one step at a time.

Recent research by sporting goods manufacturers acknowledges that weight training, with almost 40 million participants, is the single most popular type of fitness training activity in the United States. The reason for this popularity is quite simple. The results are quick and they dramatically contribute to improved strength, muscle tone, body reproportioning, appearance, and health. Unfortunately, not many books on the subject are written so that an inexperienced person can easily understand the information and use it with confidence. Terminology is often confusing, explanations are unclear, and readers are expected to understand too much information at one time. The approach taken in this book does not assume that one explanation or illustration is enough to allow readers to become knowledgeable about and skilled at weight training concepts and exercises. Instead, carefully developed procedures and drills accompany each step and provide you with ample practice and self-assessment opportunities.

This book focuses on two primary areas. First, it helps you to learn common weight training exercises that are used in a well-balanced training program. Second, it provides the knowledge you need to design your own weight training program. We begin by describing how your body will respond to weight training, the equipment you will use, and dietary and training information that is essential to success. Building on this foundation of informa-tion, basic lifting techniques and exercises are introduced, followed by more complex descriptions of exercise technique. Great care has been taken to introduce new information and higher training intensities gradually. For instance, you will start out lifting lighter training loads (weight) while you are learning proper exercise technique. Later, after you have mastered the exercises, you will progress to heavier loads. Organizing and sequencing exercises and loads in this manner offers you the best opportunity to learn without fear of injury.

Once you gain confidence, you will be ready to learn how to design your own weight training program. You will find that the practice procedures and drills included in this text are unique and provide an effective approach to explaining the content and skills of weight training. The step-by-step explanations and self-assessment activities make this book the easiest guide to weight training to follow and understand.

In addition, this new edition includes updated references and exciting variations of the previous practice and learning activities, making them more streamlined and easier to use. Also, new exercises will challenge you to develop a higher level of skill, which makes this text appropriate for those new to weight training.

Each of the 13 steps you will take is an easy transition from the one that precedes it. The first two steps of the staircase provide a solid foundation of basic skills and concepts. As you progress, you will learn to complete a basic training program in a safe and time-efficient manner. You will also learn when and how to make needed changes in program intensity. As you near the top of the staircase the climb eases, and you'll find that you have developed a sense of confidence in your weight training skills and knowledge of how to design programs that meet your specific needs. Perhaps most important, you will be pleased with how your body's appearance has changed and your fitness and energy levels have improved.

To understand how to build your training around steps 1 and 2 in this text, familiarize yourself with the concepts and directions presented in the sections that lead up to step 1. They provide information that will help you become aware of how your body reacts and adapts to weight training and the importance of proper nutrition. Questions about the proper use of machine and free-weight equipment are also answered. Finally, you will read about how to approach your training so that every minute you invest in it will count.

The Steps to Success method provides a systematic approach to executing and teaching weight training techniques and designing programs. Approach each of the steps in this way:

1. Read the explanation of what is covered in the step, why the step is important, and how to execute or perform the step's focus, which may be a basic skill, concept, approach, or combination of all three.

2. Follow the technique illustrations. They show exactly how to position your body so that you will perform each exercise correctly. The illustrations show each phase of the exercise. For each large-muscle-group exercise in the basic program, you typically will be instructed to select one exercise from three choices: one free-weight and two machine exercises.

3. Look over the missteps for common errors and ways to correct them.

4. The practice procedures and drills help you improve your skills through repetition and purposeful practice. Read the directions and the success checks for each drill and quiz. Practice accordingly and record your scores. The drills progress from easy to difficult, so be sure to achieve a satisfactory level of performance before moving on to the next drill. This sequence is designed specifically to help you achieve continual success. At the end of each step, total your scores and check your mastery of the material before moving on to the next one.

As soon as you select the exercises you will use in the basic program, you are ready to complete your first workout chart, make needed changes in the workout, and follow the basic program for a minimum of six weeks. Refer to the technique illustrations in steps 3 through 9 to evaluate your technique.

In step 10, the real fun begins. You don't have to determine which exercises to include or the number of sets and reps to perform—those decisions have already been made. All you need to do is follow the program as it is described.

Steps 11 and 12 introduce you to the logic—the whys and hows—behind the programs in step 10. These chapters include formulas and guidelines to assist you in the difficult task of determining warm-up and initial training loads and making needed adjustments to them. The helpful instructions, as well as examples and self-assessment opportunities (answers included), will prepare you for the challenge of designing your own program.

Step 13 takes you through the process of designing a program based on all of the previous steps. It is especially valuable if you are helping students design their own programs or if you are a personal trainer who designs programs for clients.

Good luck on your step-by-step journey toward developing a strong, healthy, attractive body—a journey that will be confidence-building, rich in successes, and fun!

Acknowledgments

We would like to thank several people who have influenced the development and completion of this book. Of special note is Dr. Barney Groves, coauthor of the first two editions, who provided the opportunity for Roger Earle to take on that role for this edition. We want to thank Satoshi Ochi for his assistance with the exercise illustrations. We would also like to recognize the talents of graphic artist Tara Welsch and the support and direction provided by acquisitions editor Jana Hunter and developmental editor Cynthia McEntire. Most important have been our families—Susie, Todd, and Clark Baechle and Tonya, Kelsey, Allison, Natalia, and Cassandra Earle—who have provided us with the motivation and support we needed to complete this edition.

◱ Fundamentals of Weight Training

When weight training occurs on a regular basis and is accompanied by sensible eating choices, the systems of the body change in positive ways. Muscles become stronger, become better toned, and show less fatigue with each additional session of training. The neuromuscular (nerve–muscle) system learns to work in better harmony. That is, the brain learns to selectively recruit specific muscles, and types of muscle fibers within them, to assume the loads used in weight training exercises. The neuromuscular system also improves its ability to control the speed of movement and follow the correct movement patterns that are required in each exercise.

This section will help you gain understanding of how your body responds physiologically to weight training. You will learn more about your nutritional needs, issues surrounding weight gain and weight loss, the importance of rest, and concerns about equipment and safety.

UNDERSTANDING MUSCLES

Muscle tissue is categorized into three types: smooth, skeletal, and cardiac (figure 1). In an activity like weight training, the development of skeletal muscles is of paramount importance. As shown in figure 2, skeletal muscles (sometimes referred to as striated muscles) are attached to the bone via tendons. Skeletal muscles respond to voluntary stimulation from the brain.

Although many of the more than 400 skeletal muscles are grouped together, they function either separately or in concert with others. Which and how many skeletal muscles become involved when someone performs an exercise depends on the exercise selected and the techniques used during its execution. The width of the grip or stance and the angle and path that the bar takes all affect which muscles are recruited and to what extent. Located throughout this text are illustrations and explanations of the muscle groups that are trained during the execution of specific exercises. For example, figure 3 shows the muscle, tendon, and bone relationship of the biceps muscle during the biceps curl exercise.

Isometric, concentric, and eccentric are the three different types of muscle action that can occur during weight training. The term *isometric,* or static, refers to situations in which tension develops in a muscle but no observable

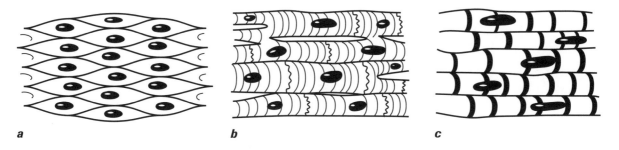

a　　　　　　　　　*b*　　　　　　　　　*c*

Figure 1　Three types of muscle tissue: *(a)* smooth; *(b)* skeletal; *(c)* cardiac.

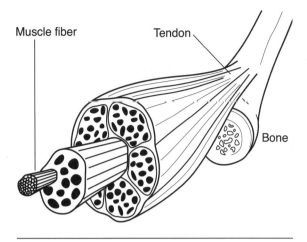

Figure 2 Tendons attach skeletal muscles to bones.

shortening or lengthening occurs. Sometimes during the execution of a repetition a sticking point is reached and a momentary pause in movement occurs. The action of the muscle(s) at this point would be described as being static. Perhaps a more understandable example would be a person attempting to push a bar off his chest during the bench press exercise when the load is too great to allow any movement upward.

Concentric muscle action occurs when tension develops in a muscle and the muscle shortens. For example, when the biceps muscle moves the barbell toward the shoulders in the dumbbell curl exercise shown in figure 4*a,* the muscle's action is described as concentric. The action of a muscle during concentric activity is also referred to as *positive work.*

The term *eccentric* is used to describe muscle action in which tension is present, but the muscle lengthens instead of shortens. Using the biceps curl as an example again, once the dumbbell begins the lowering phase (figure 4*b*), the eccentric action of the biceps controls the descent of the dumbbell. There is still tension in the biceps muscle; the difference (as compared to the concentric) is that the muscle fibers slowly lengthen to control the rate at which the dumbbell is lowered. This is referred to as *negative work* because it is performed in the direction opposite to the concentric (positive) action. The eccentric (lengthening) action, not the concentric (shortening) action, is primarily responsible for muscle soreness associated with weight training.

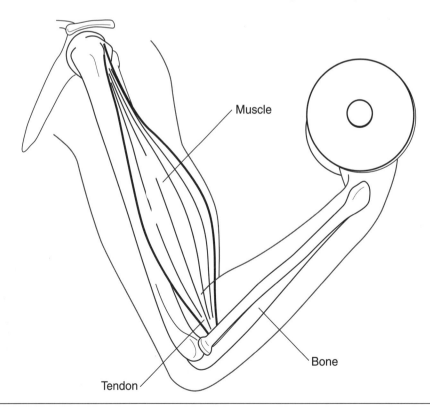

Figure 3 The biceps brachii muscle converges into a tendon and attaches to the radius bone in the forearm.

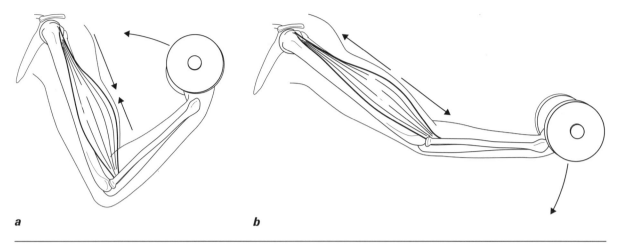

Figure 4 *(a)* During the concentric phase of the biceps curl, the muscle shortens; *(b)* during the eccentric phase, the muscle lengthens.

IMPROVEMENTS IN MUSCULAR STRENGTH

The strength you develop from weight training is influenced by neuromuscular changes (or simply neural changes) that occur through the process of learning the exercises and increasing muscle mass, and by your fiber-type composition and genetic potential.

The term *muscular strength* refers to the ability to exert maximum force during a single effort. It can be measured by determining a *one-repetition maximum effort*—referred to as a 1RM—in one or more exercises. For example, if you loaded a bar to 100 pounds (45 kilograms) and were able to complete only 1 repetition (rep) using maximum effort, your 1RM would equal 100 pounds. Strength is specific to a muscle or muscle area. This specificity concept will be discussed later.

The strength increases that occur in response to weight training have two explanations. One is associated with neural changes; the other involves increases in muscle mass. In the first case, the term *neural* refers to the nervous system working with the muscular system to increase strength. In doing so, the nerves that are attached to specific muscle fibers are taught when to transmit. Thus, an improvement in exercise technique occurs, which permits the person to lift heavier loads more efficiently and with less effort.

In the second case, through consistent training your body becomes able to recruit more

fibers and select those that are most effective in getting the job done. Thus a learning factor contributes to strength changes, some of which may be quite dramatic. This neural-learning factor explains the strength improvements seen in previously sedentary people during the first four to eight weeks of weight training.

After the first few weeks, although the neural-learning factor continues to play a role, continued gains in strength are mostly associated with increases in muscle mass. As the cross-sectional area of a muscle becomes greater because the individual fibers become thicker and stronger, so does the muscle's ability to exert force. Therefore, the neural factor accounts for early increases in strength, whereas muscle mass increases are responsible for the changes seen later.

Strength Expectations

Reported strength increases typically range from 8 to 50 percent, depending on a person's training habits and level of strength at the time of initial testing, the muscle group being evaluated, the intensity of the training program (loads, repetitions, sets, rest periods), the length of the training program (weeks, months, years), and genetic potential. The greatest improvements are seen among those who have not weight trained before and whose programs involve large-muscle exercises, heavier loads, multiple sets, and more training sessions. Unique characteristics, such as the lengths of muscles and the angles at which their tendons insert into the bone, provide mechanical advantages and disadvantages and can increase or limit an individual's strength potential.

Hearing that men are typically stronger than women should not be surprising. However, this disparity has nothing to do with the quality of muscle tissue or its ability to produce force because these are almost identical in both sexes. The quantity of muscle tissue in the average male (40 percent) versus a female (23 percent) is largely responsible for men's strength advantage. This difference also helps to explain why women are normally 43 to 63 percent weaker than men in upper-body strength and 25 to 30 percent weaker in lower-body strength.

However, to conclude that women do not have the same potential as men to gain strength is incorrect. A female can develop strength relative to her own potential, but it will not be at the same absolute strength levels achieved by males. Furthermore, weight training research studies repeatedly show that women can make dramatic improvements in strength and muscle tone without fear of developing unwanted muscle bulk. At the same time they can decrease body fat, resulting in a healthier and more attractive appearance.

Research shows that prepubescent children who participate in a well-designed, supervised weight training program can increase muscular strength above what they would experience by merely growing up. Muscular strength can increase as much as 30 to 40 percent, and children as young as age 6 have benefited from weight training. Other benefits include stronger bones, improved body composition, and an increased ability to generate power and speed.

As researchers undertake studies that involve older populations, it becomes apparent that people who follow regular exercise programs maintain their fitness levels, while those who become inactive lose about a half-pound of muscle per year during their 30s and 40s and as much as one pound per year after age 50. Herbert deVries, a well-respected researcher, contends that much of the strength loss observed in older individuals is a function of sedentary living as much as it is an outcome of the aging process.

The benefits of weight training for older people can be dramatic and positive. It can create a stronger musculoskeletal system that resists osteoporosis by enhancing bone mineral density. Plus, increased body strength reduces the incidence of degenerative diseases and improves quality of life.

In both men and women, old and young, the strength improvements that occur in response to weight training are not typically noticeable until the third or fourth week of training. The first week is usually characterized by losses in strength, perhaps due to the microtrauma (tearing down) of muscle tissue. Fatigue may also be a contributing factor. Decreases in strength performance are especially apparent during the final training session of the first week, so do not be surprised if you feel weaker toward the end of a week. Of course, you will be impressed with and excited about your strength gains, which may be as great as 4 to 6 percent per week.

Muscle-Size Increases

Exactly what accounts for muscle-size increases is not fully understood; however, factors that are often discussed are hypertrophy, hyperplasia, and genetic potential.

Muscle-size increases are most often attributed to an enlargement of existing fibers, the same fibers that were present at birth. Very thin protein strands (actin and myosin) within the fiber increase in size, creating a larger fiber. The collective effect of increases in many individual fibers is responsible for the overall muscle-size changes observed. This increase in existing fibers is referred to as *hypertrophy* (figure 5).

Although hypertrophy is the most commonly accepted explanation of why a muscle becomes larger, some studies suggest that fibers split lengthwise and form separate fibers, a theory referred to as *hyperplasia*. The splitting is thought to contribute to an increase in the size of the muscle.

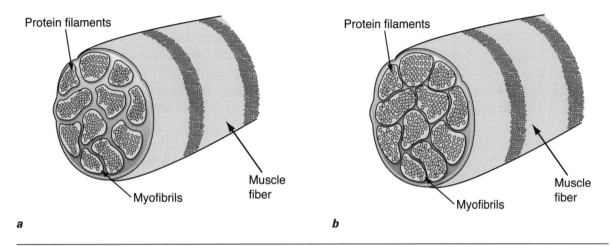

Figure 5 Muscle hypertrophy: *(a)* the muscle before training; *(b)* the muscle after training. Note the changes in the diameters of the protein filaments that constitute the myofibrils.

If one accepts hypertrophy as the process whereby existing fibers increase in size, then one must also accept that genetic limitations exist regarding the extent to which a muscle will increase in size. This is because increases are due to the thickening of fibers that already exist. Just as we know that some people are born with muscle-tendon attachments that favor force development, the same is true about the number of muscle fibers. Some people are born with a greater number of muscle fibers than others; therefore their genetic potential for hypertrophy is greater. Regardless of your genetic inheritance, your challenge is to design an effective training program and to train diligently so that you develop to your full potential.

The skeletal-muscle tissue mentioned earlier can be categorized into two basic types, each with unique capabilities and characteristics. A *fast-twitch muscle fiber* has the capacity to produce a great deal of force but fatigues quickly. Typically, its size will also increase more rapidly. Fast-twitch fibers, because of their high force capability, are recruited during weight training exercises and in athletic events that require high levels of explosive strength, such as the shot put, discus, javelin in track and field, or American football.

Slow-twitch muscle fiber is not able to exert as much force or develop it as quickly, but it is more enduring—that is, it can continue contracting for longer periods of time before fatigue sets in. Slow-twitch fibers are recruited for aerobic-oriented events such as distance running, swimming, and biking, which require less strength but greater endurance.

Not everyone possesses the same proportion of fast-twitch to slow-twitch muscle fibers. Those who possess a greater number of fast-twitch fibers have a greater genetic potential to be stronger and, therefore, to be more successful in certain strength-dependent sports or in activities like weight training. Conversely, individuals with a higher percentage of slow-twitch fibers have greater genetic potential to be successful in activities that require lower levels of strength and greater levels of endurance, such as long-distance swimming or marathon events.

IMPROVEMENTS IN MUSCULAR ENDURANCE

Muscular endurance refers to the muscle's ability to perform repeatedly with moderate loads for an extended period of time. Improvement in endurance is demonstrated by an ability to extend the period of time before muscular fatigue occurs, allowing you to perform more repetitions of an exercise. It is different from muscular strength, which is the measure of a single, all-out muscular effort. But like strength, muscular endurance is specific to the muscle or muscles involved. For instance, regularly performing a high number of reps in the biceps curl will increase endurance in the muscles in the front of the upper arm, but not in the leg muscles.

Weight training appears to produce muscular endurance improvements by reducing the number of muscle fibers involved during earlier periods of an activity, thereby leaving some in reserve should the activity continue.

The reduction in the number of fibers involved is related to strength improvements that permit a task to be undertaken using a lower percentage of effort. For example, if you had to perform a 25-pound (11-kilogram) biceps curl and had 50 pounds (22.5 kilograms) of strength in your biceps, this exercise would require 50 percent of your strength. If, however, your biceps strength increased to 100 pounds, the task would require only 25 percent of your strength—a lower percentage of effort.

IMPROVEMENTS IN CARDIOVASCULAR FITNESS

The effects of weight training on cardiovascular fitness, usually expressed as changes in oxygen uptake (the ability to transport and utilize oxygen by the muscles), have been studied by numerous researchers. It is safe to say that weight training programs that involve heavier loads, fewer repetitions, and longer rest periods between sets have a minimal effect on cardiovascular fitness. However, when they include light to moderate loads (40 to 60 percent of 1RM), a greater number of repetitions (12 or more), and very short rest periods between sets (30 to 60 seconds), a moderate (5 percent) improvement in oxygen uptake may be expected. The extent of such changes is also influenced by the intensity and length of the overall training period (weeks, months, years) as well as fitness and strength levels at the start of the program. Despite that, disre-

garding these considerations when evaluating the merits of reported cardiovascular fitness improvements attributed to weight training programs is an oversight.

The most effective way to develop cardiovascular fitness is to engage in aerobic training activities such as walking, running, swimming, cycling, or cross-country skiing. Such activities involve continuous, rhythmic movements that can be sustained for longer periods of time than anaerobic activities such as weight training. Guidelines for developing an aerobic exercise program can be found in books by Baechle and Earle (2005), Corbin and Lindsey (1997), Hoeger (1995), and Westcott and Baechle (1999), which are listed in the references section at the end of this book. A well-designed overall fitness program includes both weight training and aerobic activities.

IMPROVEMENTS IN MUSCULAR COORDINATION AND FLEXIBILITY

Despite evidence to the contrary, some people still believe that weight training will negatively affect muscular coordination and reduce flexibility. However, the feelings of heaviness in the arms and legs and numbness (loss of touch) that occur immediately after a set of repetitions are only temporary and will not reduce coordination levels. Weight training sessions most

likely will have the opposite effect. Handling and moving bars from the floor to overhead (push press), balancing the bar on your back (back squat), and evenly lifting two dumbbells (dumbbell chest fly) all contribute to improved muscular coordination.

Weight training exercises that are performed using good technique and in a controlled manner can improve strength throughout all ranges of joint motion. They will also improve flexibility, provide a better stimulus for strength development, and reduce the likelihood of injury. No evidence supports the contention that properly performed weight training exercises reduce flexibility or motor coordination.

DELAYED-ONSET MUSCLE SORENESS AND OVERTRAINING

You should not be surprised or discouraged to find that the first week or two of weight training is accompanied by some degree of muscle soreness. Although no definitive explanation exists for why we experience delayed muscle soreness, we do know that it is associated with the eccentric phase of an exercise. For example, the lowering (eccentric) phases of the biceps curl and bench press exercises can result in muscle soreness, but their upward (concentric) phases typically do not. Usually the discomfort of muscle soreness subsides after two or three days, especially if you stretch before and after training. Surprisingly, the very thing that stimulates the soreness—exercise—helps to alleviate it. Light exercise combined with stretching is ideal for speeding the recovery from muscle soreness.

Delayed-onset muscle soreness is not the same as overtraining. Overtraining is a condition in which there is a plateau or drop in performance over time. This occurs when your body does not have time to adequately recuperate from training before the next workout. Often the overtrained state is a result of overlooking the need to rest between sessions, working out too aggressively (by returning to training too soon after an illness or including too many training sessions per week), or not following recommended program guidelines.

The physical warning signs of overtraining are

- extreme muscular soreness and stiffness the day after a training session;
- a gradual increase in muscular soreness from one training session to the next;
- a decrease in body weight, especially when no effort to lose weight is made;
- an inability to complete a training session that, based on your present physical condition, is reasonable; and
- a decrease in appetite.

If you develop two or more of these symptoms, reduce the intensity, frequency, or duration of training until these warning signs subside. Preventing overtraining is more desirable than trying to recover from it.

Do the following to help prevent overtraining:

- Increase training intensity gradually.
- Alternate aggressive training weeks with less aggressive training weeks to allow for sufficient recovery between training sessions (discussed in step 12).
- Get adequate amounts of sleep.
- Eat properly.
- Make adjustments in training intensity as needed.

EATING SMART

Nutrition is the study of how carbohydrate, protein, fat, vitamins, minerals, and water provide the energy, substances, and nutrients required to maintain bodily functions during rest and exercise conditions. When a sound nutrition program is combined with regular training sessions, success is a natural outcome.

The general guidelines for a healthy diet—55 percent carbohydrate, 30 percent fat, and 15 percent protein—are appropriate for those who are weight training. Try to select foods that are complex instead of simple carbohydrates and contain unsaturated, not saturated, fat. A diet that includes appropriate amounts of fluids (six to eight glasses per day) and follows these guidelines will provide the necessary energy and nutrients to promote positive changes in strength, endurance, and muscularity.

The discussion that follows is an overview of the nutritional and dietary factors that affect your body. For more information on this topic, refer to *Nancy Clark's Sports Nutrition Guidebook, Third Edition* (2003).

Nutritional Needs

Carbohydrate is the body's primary source of energy. It provides 4 kilocalories per gram and is categorized as either complex or simple. For those who train intensely, an increased intake of complex carbohydrate is very important. Preferred sources of carbohydrate include cereal, bread, flour, grains, fruit, pasta, and vegetables (complex carbohydrates). Other sources are syrups, jellies, cakes, and honey (simple carbohydrates).

Fat provides a concentrated form of energy—9 kilocalories per gram, more than twice that of carbohydrate or protein. Fat is involved in maintaining healthy skin, insulating against heat and cold, and protecting vital organs. It is the major storage form of energy. Fat can be found in both plant and animal sources and is usually classified as saturated or unsaturated. Unsaturated fats (mono- and poly-), such as those found in olive, canola, and corn oil, are preferred because they are associated with a lower risk of developing heart disease. Common sources of saturated fat include meats (such as beef, lamb, chicken, and pork), dairy products (such as cream, milk, cheese, and butter), and egg yolks.

Proteins are the building block of all body cells. They are responsible for repairing, rebuilding, and replacing cells as well as for regulating bodily processes involved in fighting infection. If the supply of carbohydrate and fat is insufficient and the responsibility of repairing, rebuilding, and regulating metabolic functions has been met, protein can be used as a source of energy. Protein, which provides 4 kilocalories per gram, is made up of basic units called *amino acids,* which are in turn further described as essential or nonessential. Of the 20 amino acids, 8 (or 9, depending on which reference is consulted) are termed essential and must be supplied through the diet. The other 12 (or 11), the nonessential amino acids, can be produced by the body. Foods that contain all of the essential amino acids are called complete proteins. Meat, fish, poultry, eggs, milk, and cheese are sources of complete proteins. Suggested protein sources that are low in fat are milk products, lean meats, and fish. Incomplete sources of protein are breads, cereals, nuts, dried peas, and beans.

Vitamins are essential nutrients needed for many body processes. They are divided into two types, fat soluble and water soluble. Regardless of the type, vitamins do not contain energy or calories, and vitamin supplementation will not provide more energy.

Minerals function as builders, activators, regulators, transmitters, and controllers of the body's metabolic processes. Like vitamins, they do not provide calories.

Water, although it does not provide energy for activity, provides the medium for and is one of the end products of activity. Water makes up about 72 percent of the weight of muscle and represents 40 to 60 percent of a person's total body weight. Through the regulation of thirst and urine output, the body is able to keep a delicate water balance.

The Food Guide Pyramid developed by the USDA and the Department of Health and Human Services can help you choose the best foods for a healthy diet. Eating a variety of foods, increasing the amount of bread, fruit, and vegetables in your diet, and reducing the amount of fat and added sugar are recommended. Go to the USDA Web site (www.mypyramid.gov) to learn which foods and amounts are right for you based on your age, sex, and activity level.

Dieting and Weight Loss

Body composition refers to the ratio of fat weight to fat-free weight (muscles, bones, organs) that composes your body. In contrast to judging physical makeup solely on your bathroom scale

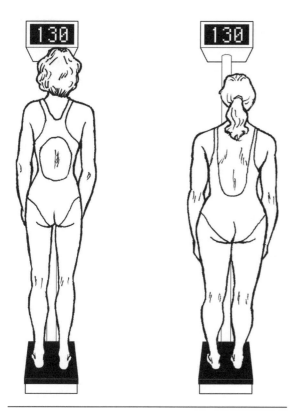

Figure 6 Two women of the same weight but with different body compositions. Note that although the woman on the left weighs the same as the woman on the right, she is much leaner.

weight, as shown in figure 6, body composition is a more accurate way to describe your health and fitness status. Two factors that have a profound effect on body composition are food intake and activity level.

Unfortunately, more than 65 million Americans are on some type of diet at any given time. Millions more are going on diets every day. Some are losing weight, but many are gaining it back. All hope to find the answer somehow. The truth is that the diets that are designed to create fast weight loss usually are not effective in helping people stay healthy and trim. In fact, many of those diets are harmful.

There are good reasons why diets typically don't work and better reasons why wise food selection plus regular exercise does work. Crash diets, in particular, are not effective because the body quickly adapts to a lower food intake by reducing its metabolic rate (the rate at which food is burned for energy). This compensatory action by the body resists the burning of fat.

When a dietary restriction results in a loss of 10 pounds, for example, the body adjusts to the restricted diet. Later, when increased food intake occurs, even though daily consumption is still less than it was before dieting, the body treats the increase as excess and stores it as fat. This yo-yo cycle of losing weight and quickly gaining it back is not only ineffective in creating a positive body appearance, but it's also unhealthy.

The weight loss experienced during the early part of a strict diet program is usually a loss of water, not fat. Many diets restrict carbohydrate intake. This reduces the water content of the body because much of the water stored in our bodies is accumulated in the process of storing carbohydrate. Weight loss due to the reduction of water stores is only temporary. Once the fluid balance is restored, a scale will not reflect the loss of body fat that was assumed to have occurred.

Also, if a female dieter consumes less than about 1,200 kilocalories a day (1,500 for a male), muscle tissue as well as fat is usually lost. The further the caloric intake dips below this amount, the more muscle tissue is lost compared to fat. So even though the dieters lose weight, they are actually fatter because the amount of body fat compared to lean body weight has increased.

The goal of a sound diet should be to reduce total body weight without losing muscle tissue. People who are on the roller coaster of dieting, gaining weight, and dieting again may be weakening their bodies every time they diet.

It appears that many overweight people justify overeating by thinking that they need more food to nourish their bodies because they are heavy. Actually, the opposite is true in many cases. Too much of their body weight is fat, which, unlike muscle, is not as metabolically active. In contrast, exercising muscles burn calories. The more muscle people have, the more energy they expend and the faster stored fat is lost. Compare two individuals who are the same height, one of whom weighs more and is in worse physical condition than the other. The lighter person has more muscle and less stored fat due to a good fitness level and requires a greater caloric intake than the less active, heavier, fatter, and less muscular person.

For many people, the most effective way to decrease excess body fat is to moderately reduce caloric intake while participating in an aerobic and weight training program. These exercise programs will burn calories and maintain or build muscle tissue, which encourages an improvement in the fat-to-muscle ratio. Aerobic activities involve the large muscles in continuous, repetitive motions such as those in cycling, swimming, walking, jogging, cross-country skiing, and rope skipping. These activities promote the greatest caloric expenditure. Golf, by comparison, is not a continuous and rhythmic activity and burns only half the calories that swimming the backstroke does for persons of the same body weight.

Weight training sessions do not normally burn as many calories as aerobic exercise sessions, but they do maintain or increase muscle mass. This is important because by adding more muscle, more calories are expended.

If you want to lose body fat, attempt to lose it at a maximum rate of 1 to 2 pounds per week. Losses greater than this result in losses of muscle tissue. A pound of fat has approximately 3,500 kilocalories, so a daily dietary reduction of 250 to 500 kilocalories will total 1,750 to 3,500 kilocalories a week. Combined with regular exercise, this decrease will promote the recommended loss of 1 to 2 pounds of fat per week and help keep it off.

Gaining Weight

Most people who exercise have no interest in gaining body weight; however, some do participate in weight training programs specifically to gain muscle. To accomplish this, an increase in caloric intake is necessary, in combination with regular training. Weight training stimulates muscle growth and increases body weight. The consumption of additional calories beyond one's daily needs provides the basis for an increase in muscle tissue. The addition of 1 pound of muscle requires 2,500 extra kilocalories. An equal increase in protein and carbohydrate (with an emphasis on complex carbohydrates) with no change in fat intake should help promote lean tissue growth and an increase in muscle size.

Note that a woman typically does not become as muscular as a man, so gaining significant body weight in response to weight training is unlikely unless she makes an effort to do so by increasing food intake and following a program designed to develop hypertrophy.

Protein Needs, Supplements, and Steroids

Although many people endorse protein, mineral, and vitamin supplementation, little research substantiates claims that it improves muscular endurance, hypertrophy, or muscular strength in people who eat nutritionally sound diets. Again and again, dietitians, exercise physiologists, and sports medicine physicians conclude that a normal diet will meet the protein dietary needs of the average person. The exception may be that an increase in carbohydrate and protein intake is appropriate for those who participate in aggressive weight training programs.

Conversations regarding supplementation are all too often accompanied by questions concerning steroids. It is human nature to look for shortcuts, especially among people who desire to make their bodies stronger, healthier, and more attractive. But there are no safe shortcuts. Anabolic-androgenic steroids, in the presence of adequate diet and training, can contribute to an increase in lean body mass; however, the harmful side effects can greatly outweigh any positive effect.

There are two forms of steroids: oral (pills) and injected (a water- or oil-based liquid that is injected using a hypodermic needle). Their potency is gauged by comparing the anabolic effects (muscle building and strength inducing) versus the androgenic effects (increased male or female secondary sex characteristics, such as increased body-hair length or density, voice lowering, and breast enlargement). This ratio is termed the *therapeutic index*.

Studies included in a position paper by the National Strength and Conditioning Association on steroid use (Stone 1993) have cited increases in muscle size and strength, but not all outcomes from their use are positive. Prolonged high dosages of steroids can lead to a long-lasting impairment of normal testosterone endocrine (natural steroid) function, a decrease in natural testosterone levels, and a potential reduction in future physical development. With a decrease in testosterone, the body cannot make gains or retain what has already been developed.

The negative health consequences of steroid use are chronic illnesses such as heart disease, liver trouble, urinary tract abnormalities, and sexual dysfunction. The immediate short-term effects include increased blood pressure, acne, testicular atrophy, gynecomastia (male breast enlargement), sore nipples, decreased sperm count, prostatic enlargement, and increased aggression. Other side effects have been well publicized, including hair loss, fever, nausea, diarrhea, nosebleeds, lymph node swelling, increased appetite, and a burning sensation during urination. Extreme psychological symptoms have also been reported, including paranoia, delusions of grandeur, and auditory hallucinations.

When steroid use is discontinued after short-term use, most side effects disappear. However, females who take steroids experience permanent deepening of the voice, facial hair, baldness, clitoral enlargement, and a decrease in breast size.

One of the most serious concerns associated with taking anabolic steroids is the development of coronary artery disease. Some researchers have reported high levels of total cholesterol, low levels of the desirable high-density lipoproteins (HDLs), and elevated blood pressure as a consequence of taking steroids, all of which are significant heart disease risk factors. However, others suggest that the cholesterol levels reported may have been present before the use of steroids began.

EQUIPMENT USE AND SAFETY

Walking into a well-equipped weight room for the first time can be confusing and somewhat intimidating. You will see machines of various sizes and shapes, short and long bars, and weight plates of varying sizes and weights with holes of different sizes (which fit onto the bars). Gaining a better understanding of equipment terminology, learning what each type of equipment is designed to do, and learning how to use each piece properly not only makes training safer but is necessary if training goals are to be achieved.

The equipment available often dictates which exercises you can include in your workouts. For example, if you do not have access to a lat machine, in step 4 you will not be able to select the lat pull-down exercise to strengthen the back muscles. Therefore, becoming familiar with the equipment and its proper use is a logical first step in starting a weight training program. This section includes information about the types, characteristics, and safe use of machine and free-weight training equipment.

Machines

Most machines in a workout facility are designed to accommodate what is referred to as a *dynamic* form of exercise—that is, exercise that involves movement. In contrast are isometric exercises, such as pulling or pushing against a fixed bar, in which no observable movement occurs. Dynamic exercises performed on weight machines challenge muscles to shorten against resistance and lengthen in a controlled manner while loaded.

Fixed-Resistance Equipment

Figure 7 shows two types of single-unit and one type of multiunit selectorized machines, which allow the user to choose a certain load. The single-unit pulley (figure 7a) and pivot-arm (figure 7*b*) types of selectorized machines are designed to isolate muscular stress on one muscle area. Multiunit machines (figure 7*c*) have two or more stations attached to their frame and allow many muscle areas to be trained by simply moving from station to station.

A closer look at the structure of these machines reveals how they are designed. The weight stack in figure 8*a* is lifted by pushing a weight arm attached to a fixed pivot point. In figure 8*b*, the weight stack is lifted by pulling down on a handle affixed to a cable–pulley arrangement. Sometimes a chain or flat belt is used in place of the cable shown in figure 8*b*.

You will notice when using fixed-resistance equipment that some movement phases require more effort than others, as though someone were changing the weight of the weight stack. What happens is that as the weight arm moves in response to being pushed or pulled, it changes the location of the weight stack (WS) in relation to the weight arm's pivot

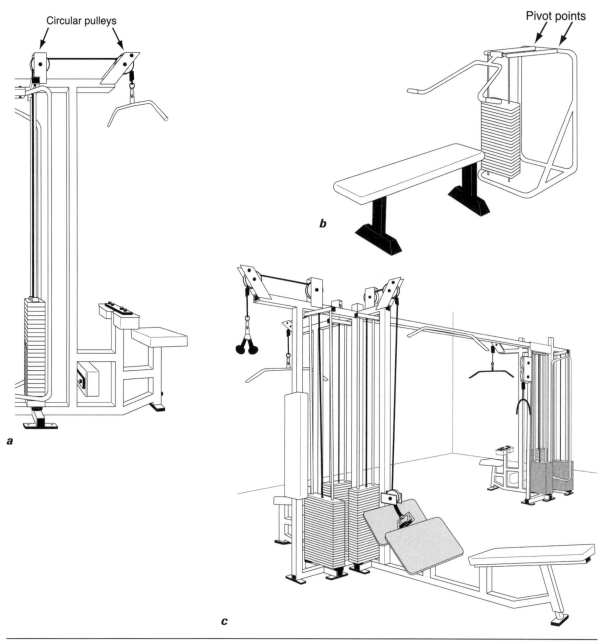

Figure 7 Weight training machines: *(a)* single-unit pulley machine; *(b)* pivot-arm type single-unit machine; *(c)* multiunit machine.

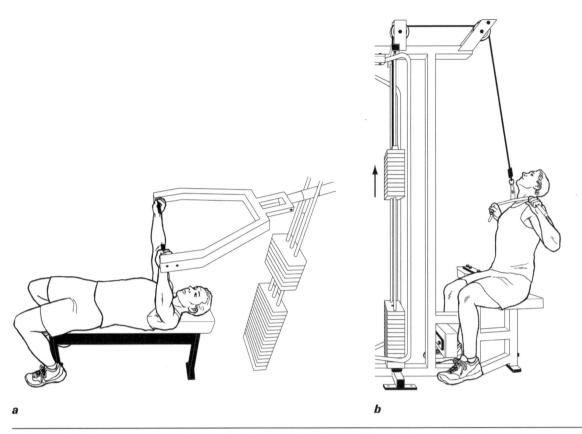

a   *b*

Figure 8 Machine structure: *(a)* pivot-arm bench press; *(b)* pulley-type lat pull-down machine.

point (PP). This is illustrated in figure 9. As the distance between the weight stack and the pivot point becomes shorter, the exercise requires less effort; as the distance becomes greater, the exercise requires more effort.

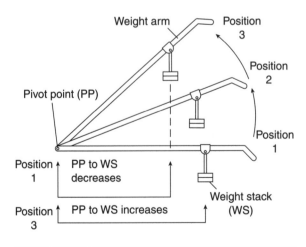

Figure 9 Fixed-resistance machine function. Note that as the weight arm is moved from position 1 to position 3, the distance from the pivot point (PP) to the weight stack (WS) decreases, making the exercise easier to complete.

Machines that feature a fixed pivot or a circular-shaped pulley design are commonly referred to as fixed-resistance machines. The limitation of this type of equipment is that the muscles are not taxed in a consistent manner throughout the range of movement in the exercise. Free weights also fall into this category and present the same limitation.

Variable-Resistance Equipment

In an effort to create a more consistent stress on muscles, some machines are designed so that during the exercise the load is decreased at the point that requires the greatest effort and increased when the least effort is needed. That is how a more consistent stress is created on the muscles as they contract throughout a repetition. These machines are referred to as variable-resistance machines (figure 10).

As shown in figure 11, when the weight (lever) arm of a variable-resistance machine moves to position 1 (which would require more

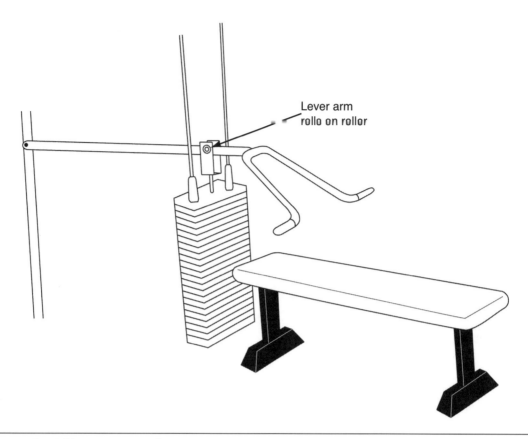

Figure 10 A variable-resistance machine.

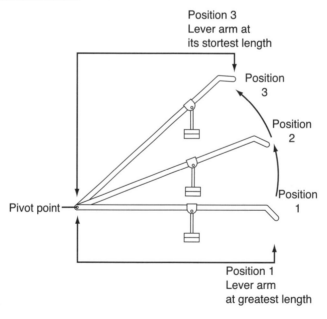

Figure 11 Variable-resistance machine function. Note that as the weight arm is moved from position 1 to position 3, the distance from the pivot point (PP) to the point of force application (FA) decreases, making the exercise harder to complete.

effort with a fixed-pivot machine), it is at its greatest length. At this length you acquire a mechanical advantage that makes it easier to perform the repetition. Conversely, when the weight arm is moved to position 3, its length is shortened, causing a mechanical disadvantage. This makes it harder to complete the repetition at this point in the exercise. There is more to understanding why changes in the length of a weight arm impose a more consistent stress throughout the entire range of an exercise, but the explanation here is sufficient to help you recognize the capabilities of variable-resistance machines.

To create a more consistent stress, variable-resistance machines may also feature a kidney-shaped wheel or cam. The effect of cam shape on the location of the weight stack is shown in figure 12. As the chain, cable, or belt tracks over the peaks and valleys of the cam, notice that the distance between the pivot point (the axle on which the cam rotates) and the weight stack changes. This variation in distance is what creates a more uniform load on the muscles. That is, at the point when the exercise becomes most difficult to perform, the distance from the weight stack to the pivot point decreases, making the load easier to move. Conversely, at the easiest point in the exercise, the distance between them increases. If you want to gain a better understanding of the principles involved in the equipment described here, consider reading Earle and Baechle (2004), Baechle and Earle (2000), Garhammer (1986), or Westcott and Baechle (1999).

Isokinetic Equipment

Not as common but also popular are isokinetic machines (figure 13). These machines are designed so that exercises (dynamic) performed on them are done at a constant speed. Unlike variable-resistance machines that involve concentric and eccentric muscle actions, isokinetic equipment involves only concentric activity. Instead of using weight stacks, these machines create resistance by using hydraulic, pneumatic, or frictional features. Control settings on these machines allow you to select movement speeds that relate to the level of resistance desired, ranging from slower speeds that require greater effort to faster speeds that require less effort as you move through the range of the exercise movement.

Isokinetic machines provide a resistance to movement that is equivalent to the force you exert. The harder you push or pull, the greater the resistance you experience; the weaker the effort, the less the resistance. The primary difference between variable-resistance and isokinetic machines is that with the former, the shape of the cam or the position of the roller dictates the effort you must exert. With

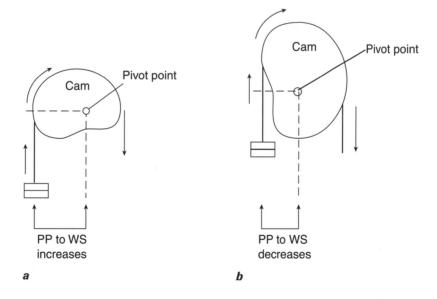

a   *b*

Figure 12 Variable-resistance cam function: *(a)* PP to WS increases; *(b)* PP to WS decreases. The cam functions similarly to the moving weight stack by varying the distance between the PP and the WS, thereby creating a more uniform stress on the muscles.

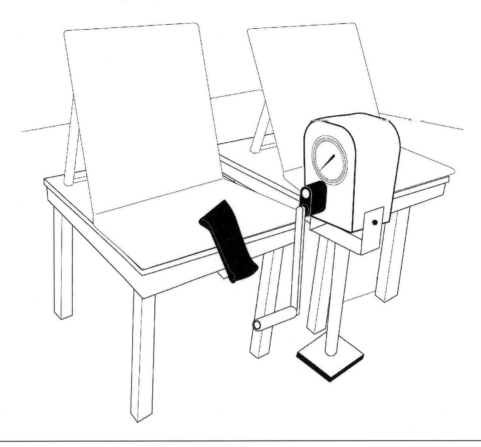

Figure 13 Isokinetic machine.

isokinetic machines, how hard you push or pull determines the effort throughout the exercise movement.

Training Precautions With Machines

You might hear that weight training machines are safer than free weights. True, they are inherently safer because the weight stacks are located away from the lifter and the bars are suspended or stationary. Thus dropped weight plates and bars are less likely to cause the same types of injuries that are associated with using free weights. The stationary nature of machines also permits safer travel to and from exercise stations (verses carrying a barbell or dumbbell). Another advantage is that if you intend to train on your own, you will not need a spotter.

Even though machines offer advantages over free weights, injuries can still occur (probably because many people who train on machines have limited experience in the weight room). A lack of experience, overconfidence when using machines, and inadequate instruction contribute to many of the muscle, tendon, and joint injuries that occur frequently in training facilities.

Following these guidelines will make training on machines safer and more productive:

1. Position yourself into the machines properly.
2. Perform exercises using the techniques described.
3. Perform exercises in a slow, controlled manner.

Before using a machine, check for frayed cables and belts, worn pulleys and chains, broken welds, loose pads, and uneven or rough movement. If any of these exist, do not use that machine until it is repaired. Adjust the levers and pads to accommodate your body size. Never place your fingers or hands between weight stacks to dislodge a selector key or adjust loads, and keep fingers and hands away from the chains, belts, pulleys, and cams.

When you are training on machines, be sure to select the correct weight. Loads that are too heavy may overstress the muscles, and those that are too light can result in injury when repetitions are performed too quickly. When getting positioned in or on a machine, assume a stable position on the seats, pads, and rollers. Fasten any seat belt securely. When choosing the appropriate load, be sure to insert the selector key all the way. Perform exercises through the full range of motion in a slow, controlled manner. Do not allow the weight stacks to bounce during the lowering phase of the exercise or to hit the top pulley during the upward phase.

Free Weights

Free-weight equipment is different in design and slightly different in function than its machine counterpart. The term *free* refers to its nonrestrictive effect on joint movement, in contrast to machines that create a predetermined movement pattern. It is this characteristic that enables a lifter to perform many exercises with only one barbell or a pair of dumbbells.

Barbells

Compare the characteristics of barbells (figure 14) with those of dumbbells (figure 17, page xxvii). On the typical barbell (figure 14a), the middle section has both smooth and knurled, or roughened, areas, with collars and locks on each end. The weight plates slide up to the collars, which stop the plates from sliding inward toward the hands. The outside locks (figure 15a) snug up to the plates and keep them from sliding off the ends. A typical bar with collars and locks weighs approximately 5 pounds (2.25 kilograms) per foot, so a 5-foot bar weighs about 25 pounds (11.25 kilograms).

The longest barbell in a weight room, an Olympic bar (figure 14b), is 7 feet (2.13 meters) long and weighs 45 pounds (20.25 kilograms) without locks. The locks vary in shape (figure 15), and their individual weight may range from less than a pound (a) to 5 pounds (b).

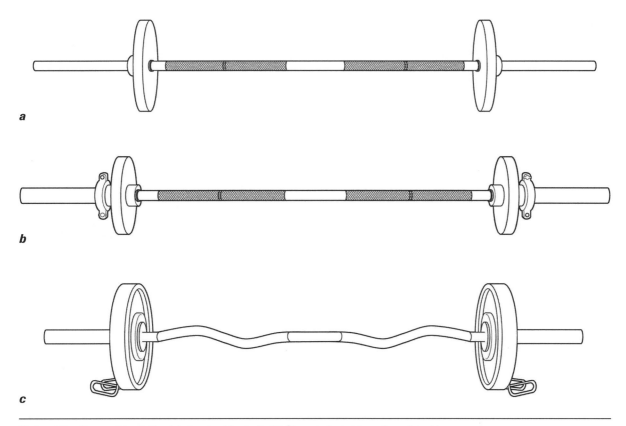

Figure 14   Types of barbells: *(a)* standard barbell; *(b)* Olympic bar; *(c)* cambered curl bar.

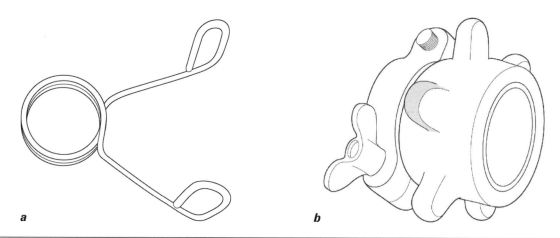

a   b

Figure 15 Locks for barbells: *(a)* spring lock (weight is usually not included in weight of bar); *(b)* Olympic lock (each weighs up to 5 pounds)

Therefore, an Olympic bar with locks can weigh as much as 55 pounds (24.75 kilograms). They have the same diameter as most bars in the weight room, except for the section between the collar and the end of the bar, where the diameter is greater. This is an important distinction to recognize when loading the bar. Only the Olympic weight plates (figure 16*a*), with larger diameter holes, will fit properly onto an Olympic bar. The plates with the smaller holes (figure 16*b*) will not fit onto it.

Another type of bar is the cambered curl bar (figure 14*c*). It has the same characteristics as the barbell, except that its curves enable the lifter to isolate stress more effectively on certain muscle groups.

Dumbbells

Dumbbells (figure 17) are similar to barbells, but they are shorter and the entire middle section of the bar between the weight plates is usually knurled (roughened). The weight of a dumbbell bar (with collars and locks, approximately 3 pounds or 1.36 kilograms) is not usually included when the weight being lifted is recorded. For example, a dumbbell with a 10-pound (4.5-kilogram) plate on each side is described as weighing 20 pounds (9 kilograms), not 23 pounds (10.4 kilograms).

Training Precautions When Using Free Weights

Using free-weight barbells and dumbbells requires higher levels of motor coordination than using machines. The freedom of movement allowed by free weights easily translates to potential injury when correct lifting, loading, and spotting techniques are not used. However, free-weight training is not dangerous; when reasonable precautions are taken, it is very safe and can be more effective than machines in strengthening joint structures.

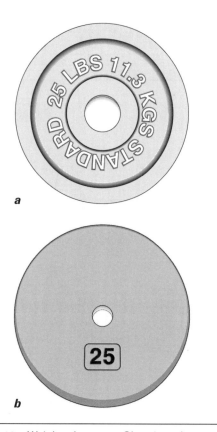

a

b

Figure 16 Weight plates: *(a)* Olympic style; *(b)* standard.

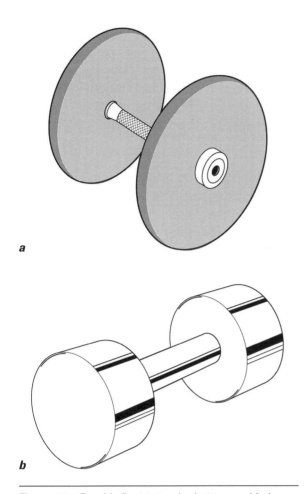

a

b

Figure 17 Dumbbells: *(a)* standard; *(b)* premolded.

As you become more familiar with the free-weight equipment, you will realize that barbells and dumbbells offer tremendous versatility—your choice of exercises is virtually unlimited. If you plan to train at home, versatility and lower cost make free weights the preferred type of equipment.

Certain precautions are advisable when using either free weights or machines. The following actions will help you avoid potentially dangerous situations and make free-weight and machine training safer.

• **Load bars properly.** Take great care to add the proper amount of weight onto bars and select the correct weight stack for machine exercises because the stress imposed on muscles due to overloading can easily cause injury. Also, if the ends of a free-weight bar are not loaded evenly, serious injury can occur to you and those nearby. Learning the weight of

the weight plates and staying alert when loading each end of a bar will help prevent these errors.

• **Lock barbells and dumbbells.** Lifting with unlocked barbells and dumbbells is dangerous. Weight plates that are not secured with locks can easily slide off the bar and land on feet or other body parts. Locks should be checked for tightness before each set of exercises. Do not assume that the last person who used the barbell or dumbbell tightened the locks. Also check to see that the collars are secure. If the locks are welded to the bar, always determine that the weld is intact.

• **Avoid backing into others.** Because of a sudden loss of balance or being unaware that anyone is near you, you may back into someone. Take care to avoid this; an untimely bump may cause injury. For example, a lifter doing a standing press could drop a barbell or dumbbell on his head; someone doing a dumbbell chest fly exercise could drop the weight into his face.

• **Be aware of extended bars.** Extended bars are those that overhang or extend outward from machines, barbells supported on racks (on the squat rack, for example) or uprights (as for the bench press), or bars held in the hands. Of special concern are bars positioned at or above shoulder height, which can cause serious facial injuries. Lat pull-down bars and free-weight barbells held at or above shoulder height are the most likely sources of such injuries. Be especially cautious around people who are performing overhead exercises or are backing out of racks with a barbell on their shoulders.

• **Store equipment properly.** Each piece of equipment in a training facility should have a particular storage location. Barbells, dumbbells, and weight plates that are not replaced in their proper locations or are left unattended are often tripped over or slipped on. Always place the equipment you use in appropriate racks and locations, whether at home or in a training facility. Care should be taken to secure weight training equipment so that children do not have access to it without proper supervision; it is dangerous for them to climb on equipment and lift plates and bars that are too heavy for them.

Another safety consideration is using a weightlifting belt (figure 18), which is commonly used by both men and women in a weight training facility. Their use may contribute to injury-free training, but they alone will not protect you from back injuries—only good technique will. Whether using one is appropriate depends on the exercise being performed and the relative amount of the load being used.

You should wear a belt in those exercises that stress the back and involve maximum or near-maximum loads. Pull it snugly into position around the waist and be sure to breath properly during its use. Performing exercises while wearing a belt that's too tight or while not breathing properly can contribute to dizziness, blackouts, and cardiovascular complications.

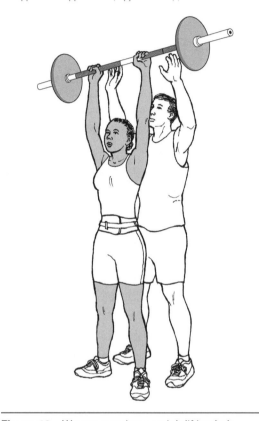

Figure 18   Woman wearing a weightlifting belt.

Equipment Drills

A logical starting point for novice trainees is to becoming familiar with the types of weight training equipment and their safe use. This includes being able to identify what the equipment is designed to do, knowing how to use it, and determining whether it is in good working order. It is unwise to train on any piece of equipment until these things are known. The following drills test your understanding of the concepts covered; modify them as needed to fit your situation.

Equipment Drill 1.   *What Equipment Is Available?*

Survey the equipment in your facility. Which types do you recognize? Place a check mark next to the equipment you observe.

Machine Equipment

1. Fixed resistance ___

2. Variable resistance

    a. Pivot ___

    b. Cam ___

3. Isokinetic ___

Free-Weight Equipment

1. Standard bar ___

2. Olympic bar ___

3. Cambered curl bar ___

4. Dumbbells ___

Equipment Drill 2. *Equipment Safety Review*

Safety is so important that you need to get in the habit of checking the equipment each time you train. Walk through your facility and check the status of the equipment using the checklists shown in figure 19. Repeat this process each time you work out. A common source of litigation involves equipment that was not in good working order when the person was injured.

Machine Equipment Safety Checklist

Mark each item as it is completed.

Before each training session:

_____ Check for frayed cables, belts, pulleys, worn chains, loose pads.

_____ Check for proper lever and seat adjustments.

During each training session:

_____ Assume a stable position on seats and pads.

_____ Fasten belts securely (if applicable).

_____ Insert selector keys/pins properly.

_____ Perform exercises in a slow, controlled manner.

a

Free-Weight Equipment Safety Checklist

Mark each item as it is completed.

Before performing each set:

_____ Check for integrity of collar welds.

_____ Check for tightness of collars and locks.

_____ Check for correct load on both ends of the bar.

During each training session:

_____ Avoid walking into bars that extend outward.

_____ Avoid walking near people who are performing overhead exercises.

_____ Avoid backing into others.

_____ Perform exercises in a slow, controlled manner.

After each training session:

_____ Return equipment to its proper location.

b

Figure 19 Safety checklists: *(a)* machine equipment; *(b)* free-weight equipment.

WARM-UP AND COOL-DOWN ACTIVITIES

Because of the demands that training places on muscles and joints, warming up properly before each session is important. Warm-up activities such as brisk walking or jogging in place for about 5 minutes, followed by an appropriate stretching routine, helps to physically and mentally prepare you to train. Stretching also improves flexibility (the ability to move joints through a full range of motion), and in doing so may help prevent injury.

Go through a warm-up activity and then follow the series of static (held) stretching positions described and illustrated here. Be sure to move slowly into the stretched positions, without bouncing. The stretches presented involve major joints and muscle groups, especially the less flexible muscles of the backs of the legs, the upper and low back, and the neck. Refer to the muscle illustrations shown in step 2 to learn their names and locations.

Include these stretching exercises prior to and immediately after each training session. Brisk walking or jogging plus stretching increases blood and muscle temperatures, enabling muscles to contract and relax with greater ease. Stretching afterward helps speed recovery from muscle soreness. Most important, a proper warm-up helps to prevent injuries during training. Hold each of the stretching positions for at least 10 seconds and repeat them two or three times.

Chest and Shoulders

Grasp your hands together behind your back and slowly lift them upward (figure 20), or simply reach back as far as possible if you are not able to grasp your hands. For an additional stretch, bend at the waist and raise your arms higher.

Upper Back, Shoulder, and Arm

With your right hand, grasp your left elbow and pull it slowly across your chest toward your right shoulder. You will feel tension along the outside of your left shoulder and arm (figure 21). Repeat with the other arm. You can vary

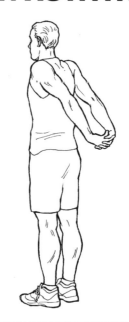

Figure 20   Chest and shoulder stretch.

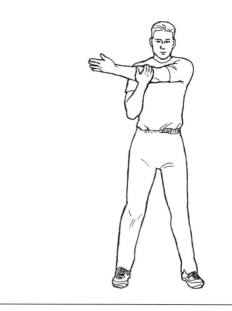

Figure 21   Upper back, shoulder, and arm stretch.

this stretch by pulling the arm across and down over your chest and upper abdomen.

Shoulder and Triceps (Back of Upper Arm)

Bring both arms overhead and hold your left elbow with your right hand. Allow your left arm to bend at the elbow, and let your left hand rest against the back of your right shoulder or upper back. Slowly pull with your right hand to move the left elbow behind your head until you feel a stretch (figure 22). Repeat with the other arm.

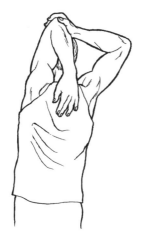

Figure 22 Shoulder and triceps stretch.

Back and Hip

Sit with your right leg straight. Bend your left leg and cross your left foot over your right leg, placing it next to the outside of your right knee with the sole flat on the floor. Then twist your body to the left and push against the outside of your upper left thigh, just above the knee, with your right elbow. Use your right elbow to keep this leg stationary as you perform the stretch. Next, place your left hand behind your buttocks, slowly turn your head to look over your left shoulder, and rotate your upper body toward your left hand and arm (figure 23). You should feel tension in your low back, hips, and buttocks. Repeat with the other leg.

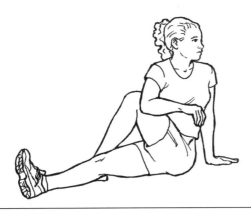

Figure 23 Back and hip stretch.

Back, Hamstring, and Inner Thigh

While seated on the floor, straighten your right leg. Bend your left leg and place the sole of your left foot so that it is slightly touching the inside of your right knee. Bend forward from the hips slowly, sliding the palms of your hands on your thighs toward your right ankle until you feel tension in the back of your right thigh (figure 24). Be sure to keep the toes of your right foot pointing up while your ankle and toes are relaxed. Perform the same stretch with the left leg.

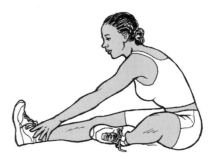

Figure 24 Back, hamstring, and inner-thigh stretch.

Quadriceps

This stretch is performed in the standing position. Using a wall or stationary object for balance, grasp your right foot with your left hand and pull so that your heel moves back toward your buttocks (figure 25). You should feel tension along the front of your right thigh. Repeat with your left leg and right hand.

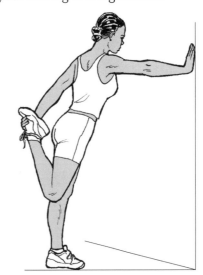

Figure 25 Quadriceps stretch.

Calves

Stand facing a wall or stationary object about 2 feet away. With your feet together and knees straight, lean forward. Apply a stretch on your calves by slowly moving your hips toward the wall. Be sure to keep your heels on the floor and your back straight (figure 26). You can stretch another muscle area of the calf by allowing the knees to flex slightly while in this same position.

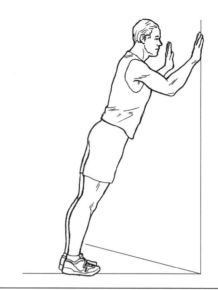

Figure 26   Calf stretch.

Warm-Up and Cool-Down Drill.   *Review*

Before performing any of the exercises in steps 3 through 9, take time to review and practice the warm-up and cool-down exercises described here. Start with a brisk walk or jog in place for 5 minutes, then perform the appropriate stretching exercises for the major joints and muscle groups: the chest and shoulders; upper back, shoulder, and arm; shoulder and triceps; back and hip; back, hamstring, and inner thigh; quadriceps; and calves.

Hold each stretch for at least 10 seconds and repeat two to three times. Avoid bouncing! Once you start training, remember to repeat two to three sets of each stretch after your workout as well.

Success Check

- Always warm up before stretching and after training.
- Move slowly into the stretches.
- Use static (versus ballistic) stretches.

RESOURCES

Little doubt remains that weight training has gained universal acceptance as an expedient method of improving the health, performance, and appearance of millions of people. The mythology surrounding weight training's dark ages has given way to mounting scientific evidence that encourages its use and an enlightened understanding of its benefits. A longtime advocate of weight training and a key player in creating interest in and support for it is the National Strength and Conditioning Association (NSCA).

A nonprofit educational association of more than 29,000 members from more than 52 countries, the NSCA stands alone as the world's recognized clearinghouse for accurate and up-to-date weight training information. Its two publications—*Essentials of Strength Training and Conditioning, Second Edition,* and *NSCA's Essentials of Personal Training*—remain the most comprehensive books on strength and conditioning and personal training produced to date. Additionally, the NSCA offers many educational programs, workshops, professional services, and journals, all at reduced rates for its members.

For information about the NSCA, go online to www.nsca-lift.org, call 719-632-6722 (800-815-6826 toll free), email nsca@nsca-lift.org, or contact the national headquarters at 1885 Bob Johnson Drive, Colorado Springs, CO 80906.

◲ Conversion Chart

To convert pounds to kilograms, multiply pounds by .453593. For an estimate, use .4536. In this chart, numbers are rounded off by reducing to the nearest quarter. For example, 185 multiplied by .453593 equals 83.9147. The kilograms are given here as 83.75 rather than 84.00. To convert kilograms to pounds, multiply kilograms by 2.2046. For a quick estimate, use 2.2.

Pounds to kilograms				Kilograms to pounds			
Pounds	Kilograms	Pounds	Kilograms	Kilograms	Pounds	Kilograms	Pounds
2.5	1.00	205	92.75	2.5	5.5	95.0	209.25
5	2.25	210	95.25	5.0	11.0	97.5	214.75
10	4.50	215	97.50	7.5	16.5	100.0	220.25
15	6.75	220	99.75	10.0	22.0	102.5	225.75
20	9.00	225	102.00	12.5	27.5	105.0	231.25
25	11.25	230	104.25	15.0	33.0	107.5	236.75
30	13.50	235	106.50	17.5	38.5	110.0	242.5
35	15.75	240	108.75	20.0	44.0	112.5	248.0
40	18.00	245	111.00	22.5	49.5	115.0	253.5
45	20.25	250	113.25	25.0	55.0	117.5	259.0
50	22.50	255	115.50	27.5	60.5	120.0	264.5
55	24.75	260	117.75	30.0	66.0	122.5	270.0
60	27.00	265	120.00	32.5	71.5	125.0	275.5
65	29.25	270	122.25	35.0	77.0	127.5	281.0
70	31.75	275	124.50	37.5	82.5	130.0	286.5
75	34.00	280	127.00	40.0	88.0	132.5	292.0
80	36.25	285	129.25	42.5	93.5	135.0	297.5
85	38.50	290	131.50	45.0	99.0	137.5	303.0
90	40.75	295	133.75	47.5	104.5	140.0	308.5
95	43.00	300	136.00	50.0	110.0	142.5	314.0
100	45.25	305	138.25	52.5	115.5	145.0	319.5
105	47.50	310	140.50	55.0	121.25	147.5	325.0
110	49.75	315	142.75	57.5	126.75	150.0	330.5
115	52.00	320	145.00	60.0	132.25	152.5	336.0
120	54.25	325	147.25	62.5	137.75	155.0	341.5
125	56.50	330	149.50	65.0	143.25	157.5	347.0
130	58.75	335	151.75	67.5	148.75	160.0	352.5
135	61.00	340	154.00	70.0	154.25	162.5	358.0
140	63.50	345	156.25	72.5	159.75	165.0	363.75
145	65.75	350	158.75	75.0	165.25	167.5	369.25
150	68.00	355	161.00	77.5	170.75	170.0	374.75
155	70.25	360	163.25	80.0	176.25	172.5	380.25
160	72.50	365	165.50	82.5	181.75	175.0	385.75
165	74.75	370	167.75	85.0	187.25	177.5	391.25
170	77.00	375	170.00	87.5	192.75	180.0	396.75
175	79.25	380	172.25	90.0	198.25	182.5	402.25
180	81.50	385	174.50	92.5	203.75		
185	83.75	390	176.75				
190	86.00	395	179.00				
195	88.25	400	181.25				
200	90.50						

Understanding the Basics of Lifting and Training

Thus far you have gained knowledge of the physiology behind weight training and of the equipment you will use. Now is an ideal time to master fundamental lifting skills that you will use in every workout. The lifting techniques described in this step can be applied to everyday physical tasks at home and work, thus decreasing the likelihood of injuring the low back. You will also learn how to breathe correctly while weight training and how to use and be a spotter for free-weight exercises.

Correctly performing basic lifting skills avoids placing excessive stress on muscles, tendons, ligaments, bones, and joints, decreasing the likelihood of injury. One of the most common debilitating conditions is low back pain, a condition that afflicts more than 300,000 people every year and results in an average of seven days of missed work per person. Proper lifting skills also produce quicker training results because muscles can be properly stressed and stimulated more effectively.

Learning to breathe properly is an important part of developing good fundamental lifting skills as well. Proper breathing helps prevent dizziness or blackouts, which can lead to life-threatening circumstances.

The fundamentals learned in this step can be applied to all exercises and spotting procedures described in this text. As you learn basic lifting and spotting skills, consider using a dowel stick (like a broom handle), a very light bar, or the lightest weight plate on a machine.

TRAINING FUNDAMENTALS

Before you learn proper lifting technique, let's review some fundamentals of training that you need to know in order to train safely, efficiently, and effectively. The essentials of productive training that are outlined here are reiterated and discussed as needed in the rest of the steps of this book.

• **Train on a regular basis.** The old adage "Use it or lose it" is unfortunately true when it comes to maintaining cardiovascular efficiency, muscular strength and endurance, flexibility, and lean muscle mass. The body is unlike any machine yet to be developed. Its efficiency improves with use, in contrast to machines, and it deteriorates with disuse. Sporadic training slows down goal attainment and has been the downfall of many beginning weight trainees who started out with good intentions.

All too often, the demise of a regular training program begins with one missed workout and ends with missing many more. Each time a training session is missed, goals for improving fitness, strength, and appearance move further out of reach. Working out regularly is important because decreases in training status begin to occur after 72 hours of no training.

• **Gradually increase training intensity.** The body adapts to the stresses of weight training when training occurs on a regular basis and when its intensity increases progressively over a reasonable period of time. Conversely, when the intensity of training is haphazard, the body's ability to adapt and become stronger and more enduring is compromised. The dramatic improvements observed in response to training do not happen under these conditions, and the excitement that prompts you to continue training is no longer present. As excitement dwindles, attending training sessions becomes more difficult and improvements become nonexistent. Muscle soreness does not go away, discouraging your enthusiasm for training even more.

• **Be willing to persevere.** To maximize the time spent in training, you must learn to push yourself to the uncomfortable point of muscle failure during many of your sets (after you know how to properly perform the exercise, of course). You must be willing to persevere through the discomfort (not pain) that accompanies reaching this point.

Believing that weight training can make dramatic changes in your health and physique—which it can—is essential to making the commitment to train hard and regularly. Typically, you will feel the difference in muscle tone (firmness) immediately. Strength and endurance changes become noticeable after the second or third week. Be prepared, however, for variations in performance during the early stages of training, and do not become discouraged if one workout does not produce the outcomes of a previous one.

Your brain is going through a learning curve as it tries to figure out which muscles to recruit (call into action) for specific movements in each exercise. Your neuromuscular system (brain, nerves, and muscles) is learning to adapt to the stimulus of training. Be patient! This period is soon followed by significant gains in muscle tone and strength and decreased muscle soreness. This is an exciting time in your program! At this point your attitude dictates the magnitude of the future gains you will experience.

• **Strive for quality reps.** Many people seem to believe that doing more repetitions in an exercise is synonymous with improvement, regardless of the technique used. The speed with which repetitions are performed is a very important factor in your ability to execute quality reps.

In an advanced weight training exercise program designed to develop power, explosive exercise movements are required. However, in a beginning program, slow, controlled movements are desired. Exercises must be performed slowly enough to permit full extension and flexion at a joint. In the biceps curl, for example, the elbow should be fully extended and then fully flexed. Jerking, slinging, and using momentum are not recommended ways to complete a repetition.

Remember that the quality of the execution should be more important than the number of repetitions performed, especially when the goal is improved flexibility. Other recommendations concerning proper exercise execution are provided in steps 3 through 9.

• **Always warm up and cool down.** Workouts should always begin with some warm-up exercises so that the muscles are better prepared to meet the challenges presented by the exercises. A cool-down period will allow your muscles to recover and offers an excellent opportunity to work on flexibility. Guidelines for appropriate warm-up and cool-down exercises were presented in Fundamentals of Weight Training (see page xxxi).

• **Eat smart.** Nutrition is a key factor. It makes no sense to train hard if you are not eating nutritionally sound meals. Poor nutrition in itself can reduce strength, muscular endurance, and muscle hypertrophy. Because training puts great demands on your body, you needs nutrients to encourage adaptation and promote gains. To neglect this aspect of your training is an oversight if you are serious about improving. See Fundamentals of Weight Training, pages xvii to xxi, for a more detailed discussion of nutrition.

• **Build days of rest into your program.** The intervening days of rest in your training program are important in terms of gaining strength, muscular endurance, and size. To train on consecutive days without the rest that allows the body to recuperate may result in injury, strand you on a training plateau, or cause a drop in performance. Properly timed rest is as important to your strength gains as training on a regular basis.

• **Obtain medical clearance.** Weight training may be an inappropriate activity if you have (or have a history of) joint problems such as arthritis or surgery, respiratory conditions such as asthma, or cardiovascular problems such as hypertension, heart arrhythmias, or heart murmurs. The implications of such conditions must be addressed before you develop an exercise program and certainly before exercise begins. Carefully consider the questions presented in figure 1.1. If you answer yes to any of them, consult a physician prior to beginning a training program.

• **Use proper training-room etiquette.** Just like participants in tennis, bowling, golf, and other sports recognize certain rules and courtesies, you should understand the rules that apply to weight training. Some are related to safety; others are matters of courtesy. When everyone in the training room abides by the following

Consult a physician before beginning a weight training program if you answer yes to any of the following questions.

Yes   No

___   ___   Have you had surgery or experienced bone, muscle, tendon, or ligament problems, especially back or knee problems, that might be aggravated by an exercise program?

___   ___   Are you over age 50 (female) or 45 (male) and unaccustomed to exercise?

___   ___   Do you have a history of heart disease?

___   ___   Has a doctor ever told you that your blood pressure was too high?

___   ___   Are you taking any prescription medications, such as those for heart problems or high blood pressure?

___   ___   Have you ever experienced chest pain, spells of severe dizziness, or fainting?

___   ___   Do you have a history of respiratory problems such as asthma?

___   ___   Is there a physical or health reason not already mentioned why you should not follow a weight training program?

Figure 1.1 Medical clearance checklist.

Reprinted, by permission, from T. R. Baechle and R. W. Earle, 1995, *Fitness Weight Training* (Champaign, IL: Human Kinetics), 24.

rules and courtesies, training experiences for all will be safer and more enjoyable.

- Return equipment to its original location.
- Wipe down equipment after using it.
- Do not perform overhead exercises near someone who is performing exercises in a supine position, such as bench press, dumbbell chest fly, or abdominal crunch.

- Avoid performing exercises close to someone else.
- Offer to let others "work in" (use the same piece of equipment) between your sets.
- Offer to spot others if you have the skill and strength to do so.
- Do not monopolize equipment.
- Place barbells and dumbbells on the floor instead of dropping them.

CORRECT LIFTING TECHNIQUE

The techniques of lifting involve focusing on

1. acquiring a good grip,
2. having a stable position from which to lift,
3. keeping the object being lifted close to the body, and
4. using your legs, not your back, when lifting a weight or bar off the floor.

Gripping the Bar

Two things to consider when establishing a grip are the type of grip used and the positioning of the hands on the bar (where on the bar and how far apart they are from each other). The grips that may be used to lift a bar off the floor are the *overhand,* or *pronated,* grip; the *underhand,* or *supinated,* grip; and the *alternated* grip. Palms are face down, or away, in the overhand grip (figure 1.2*a*), and the thumbs face each other. In the underhand grip (figure 1.2*b*) palms are facing upward, or toward you, while the thumbs face away from each other. The alternated grip (figure 1.2*c*), sometimes referred to as a *mixed grip,* involves having one hand in an underhand grip and the other in an overhand grip. In the alternated grip, the thumbs point in the same direction. (It does not matter which hand is positioned overhand or underhand in the alternated grip.) All of these are called *closed grips,* meaning that the fingers and thumbs are wrapped (closed) around the bar.

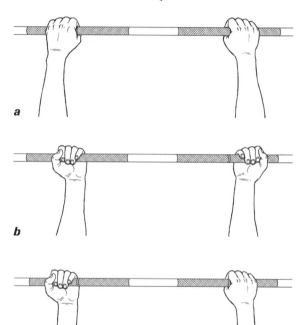

Figure 1.2 Closed bar grips: *(a)* overhand; *(b)* underhand; *(c)* alternated.

An *open grip* (figure 1.3), sometimes referred to as a *false grip,* is one in which the thumbs do not wrap around the bar. It is very dangerous because the bar can easily roll out of your hands onto your head, face, or foot, causing severe injury. Always use a closed grip!

Figure 1.4 shows several grip widths used in weight training. In some exercises the width of the grip places the hands approximately at shoulder-width and equidistant from the weight plates. This is referred to as the *common grip.*

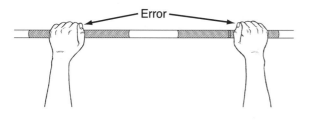

Figure 1.3 The open grip is an incorrect technique. Using it increases the risk of injury.

Some exercises require a narrow grip, others a wider grip. Learn the proper width for each exercise, as well as where to place the hands so that the bar is held in a balanced position. Improperly gripped bars with weight plates that are not locked can result in the weights falling or being catapulted off the ends of the bar, causing serious injury. Becoming familiar with the smooth and knurled areas of the bar and where the hands should be placed will help you establish a balanced grip. Note that the common grip is used later in explaining proper lifting techniques.

Lifting the Bar Off the Floor

Several phases must be followed to safely lift a bar off the floor. Some exercises require you to lift the bar from the floor just to the front

of your thighs (see figure 6.1*a,* page 70); for other exercises, you will need to lift the bar up to your shoulders in two bar movements to get into the initial or preparatory body position to perform an exercise (for example, see the standing press exercise in step 5, page 56). Some exercises consist entirely of lifting the bar off the floor (see step 9 for descriptions of total-body exercises).

This section describes four phases: a beginning or starting phase, two movement phases, and a final phase. The beginning phase has no movement; in it, you get into the correct initial body position for the exercise. During the final phase you safely return the bar to the floor.

Preparatory Lifting Position

Take hold of the bar using an overhand grip, and position the hands outside of the legs. Now move into the correct preparatory position shown in figure 1.5. Shuffle your feet toward the bar so that your shins are almost touching it. Positioning the bar close to the shins keeps the weight being lifted closer to the body during the lifting/pulling action, enabling you to exert a more effective force with your legs (and avoiding straining your low back). A key concept to remember is that a stable lifting position strategically positions the leg muscles to effectively contribute in lifting the barbell.

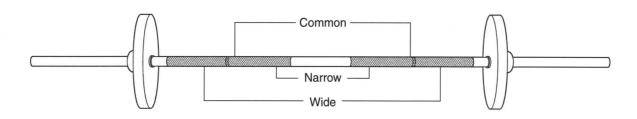

Figure 1.4 Grip widths: common, narrow, and wide.

| Figure 1.5 | Preparatory Lifting Position |

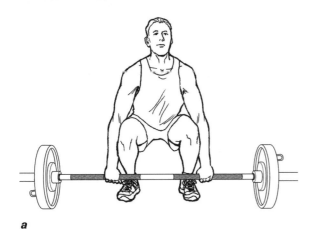

a

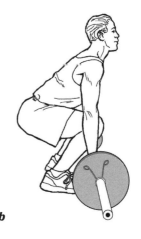

b

FRONT VIEW

1. Grip slightly wider than shoulder width
2. Feet are shoulder-width apart
3. Feet are flat on floor, toes pointed slightly outward
4. Hips are low—"gorilla" position

SIDE VIEW

1. Arms are straight, shoulders are over or slightly forward of bar
2. Head is up, eyes are focused straight ahead throughout exercise
3. Back is flat and tensed
4. Scapulae (shoulder blades) are pulled toward each other
5. Chest is held high

Establish a stable position by placing your feet flat on the floor, shoulder-width apart or slightly wider, with the toes pointing slightly outward. A wide stance, or base of support, provides greater stability and a more balanced lifting position. Establishing a stable position is especially important when performing over-head exercises with dumbbells or a barbell. It is also important when performing machine exercises that require the positioning of the feet on the floor, or the head, torso, hips, and legs on or against equipment.

Think of the body position of a gorilla! Believe it or not, this is an ideal position for lift-ing a barbell off the floor. To get into this posi-tion, grasp the bar as previously described and simultaneously straighten your elbows as you lower your hips. Now position your shoulders over or slightly ahead of the bar while keeping the head up. Focus your eyes straight ahead. Your back should be in a flat or slightly arched

position. Establish a chest-out-and-shoulders-back position by pulling the scapulae (shoulder blades) toward each other. Avoid the rounded back position shown in figure 1.6.

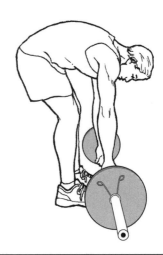

Figure 1.6 Do not round the back when lifting the bar from the floor. This puts unnecessary stress on the low back.

Often one or both heels will lift up when you move into the low position shown in figure 1.5, causing you to step forward to catch your balance. If this happens, work on drill 2, preparation position (see page 13).

Also, a proper head position, with the eyes looking straight ahead, is critical to maintaining proper body positioning. If there is a mirror available, watch yourself as you move into the low preparatory position. Does your back stay in a flat position, and do your heels stay in contact with the floor? Say these things to yourself: "Keep the bar close," "The hips stay low as the legs straighten," and "The back remains flat throughout the lifting." Keeping your head upright and your eyes looking straight ahead will help you accomplish these things. Get a mental picture of the head, shoulder, back, and hip positions. The most important things to remember are to keep the barbell, dumbbell, or weight plate as close to you as possible and to use your leg muscles, not your back! In preparation for pulling, breathe in to stabilize your upper torso.

From Floor to Thighs

During the floor-to-thigh phase shown in figure 1.7, pull the bar upward in a slow, controlled manner. Do not jerk the bar off the floor. Once it reaches the midthigh level, exhale. At this height, the barbell may be placed in a rack or handed to a partner. Bringing the bar to this height is also the first phase of a movement that takes the bar to a position at the shoulders in preparation for the standing press exercise described in step 5.

Figure 1.7   **Floor-to-Thigh Phase**

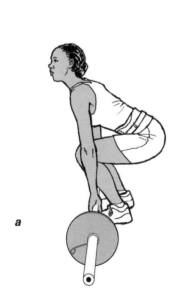
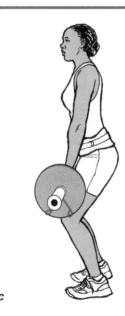

a   b   c

POSITION

1. Inhale before pulling
2. Pull in a slow, controlled manner
3. Keep the back flat

LIFT

1. Begin to straighten knees while hips stay low
2. Keep elbows straight
3. Keep bar close to shins, knees, and thighs

STRAIGHTEN

1. Keep shoulders over the bar as knees straighten
2. Exhale when bar reaches midthigh

Misstep

Your upward pull is not smooth.

Correction

Straighten your elbows before pulling, and pull slowly.

Misstep

Your hips rise first when pulling.

Correction

This movement puts stress on your back rather than on your legs. Your knees are straightening too soon! Think, "I lead my upward movement with my shoulders, not my hips." This will enable you to use your legs instead of your back to do the lifting.

If your heels rise during the floor-to-thigh phase, you have too much weight on the balls of your feet. You also may be leaning too far forward. Sit back into the low position and concentrate on putting more weight on your heels.

From Thighs to Shoulders

If you need to lift the barbell to your shoulders, continue pulling up on the bar. Do not allow the bar to slow down or rest on your thighs, and do not exhale yet. Instead, continue pulling the bar so that it brushes against your thighs as you pull upward (figure 1.8a). This keeps the bar close and reduces stress on the low back. As your knees straighten, your hips should move forward quickly.

Misstep

The bar stops on your thighs.

Correction

The pull from the floor to your shoulders should be continuous. Do not allow yourself to pause or stop the bar at your thighs.

Misstep

The bar swings away from your thighs and hips.

Correction

Concentrate on pulling the bar up straight and keeping it in close to your thighs and hips.

Follow this movement phase with a rapid shoulder shrug using the trapezius muscles between the neck and shoulders (figure 1.8b). Exhale immediately after the shrug. At the end of the shrugging motion, flex your elbows and move them upward and out to the sides to continue pulling the bar as high as possible (figure 1.8c).

Figure 1.8   Thigh-to-Shoulder Phase

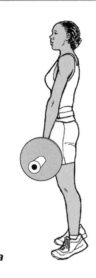

a

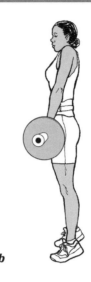

b

JUMP

1. Bar brushes middle or tops of thighs
2. Keep bar close to body as hips drive forward
3. Keep elbows straight
4. Straighten legs and hips completely

SHRUG

1. Rapidly shrug the shoulders
2. Shrug as high as possible
3. Keep elbows straight

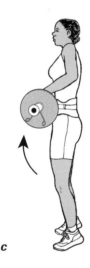

c

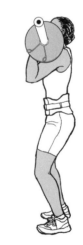

d

PEAK

1. Flex elbows and move them upward and sideways
2. Keep elbows above wrists
3. Continue pulling bar to highest point

CATCH

1. Rotate elbows down under, then up in front of bar
2. Catch (rack) bar on fronts of shoulders
3. Flex knees and hips to absorb bar's impact
4. Move upper arms to be parallel to floor
5. Gain balance and stand up

Misstep

Your elbows flex too soon.

Correction

Wait until your shrug is at its highest point before flexing your elbows.

Once the bar reaches its highest point, rack (catch) the bar on the front of your shoulders by rotating your elbows down under and then up in front of the bar as it touches your shoulders and clavicle (figure 1.8*d*). While catching the bar, simultaneously flex the knees and hips partially to help absorb the force of the bar's impact on your shoulders. After reaching a balanced position with your upper arms parallel to the floor, finish the upward phase by standing up straight.

From Shoulders to Floor

When lowering the bar (or any other heavy object) to the floor, use what you have learned about establishing a stable position, keeping the bar close and the back flat, and using your legs instead of your back to lower the bar. Also remember to lower it to the floor in a slow, controlled manner.

With the bar at shoulder height as shown (figure 1.9*a*), allow its weight to slowly pull your arms to a straightened position (figure 1.9*b*), which should briefly place the bar in a resting position on your thighs. Your hips and knees should be flexed so that as the bar touches your thighs, its weight is absorbed momentarily before you lower it to the floor. Remember to keep your head up and your back flat throughout the bar's return to the floor (figure 1.9*c*).

| Figure 1.9 | Shoulders-to-Floor Phase |

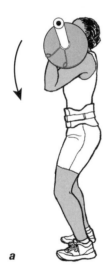
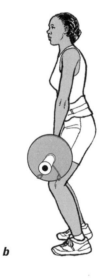
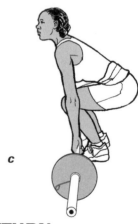

a　　　　　　*b*　　　　　　*c*

LOWER

1. Unrack the bar
2. Lower bar to thighs first
3. Flex hips and knees to absorb weight

PAUSE

1. Keep back flat or slightly arched
2. Keep shoulders back
3. Keep bar close to thighs, knees, shins

RETURN

1. Lower bar to floor, under control

Misstep

The bar does not pause at your thighs.

Correction

Visualize the downward phase as a two-count movement, "one" to the thigh, "two" to the floor.

 Misstep

Your hips remain high as you lower the bar from thigh height to the floor.

Correction

This position is stressful on the back! Once the bar reaches the thighs, squat down to lower it while keeping an upright, flat back position.

BREATHING

The best time to exhale in most exercises is during the sticking point, or the most difficult point in a repetition. Inhalation should occur during the relaxation phase, or easiest point in a repetition. For example, in the upward movement of the biceps curl, exhalation should occur when the forearms are parallel with the floor (the most difficult point). Inhalation should occur as the bar is being lowered (the easiest point). In exercises in which upper-torso stabilization is needed to help maintain a correct lifting position, such as in the back squat (step 7) or hang clean (step 9), breathing should occur at the end of the sticking point. For exercises and drills shown in steps 2 through 9, remember to breathe out through the sticking point!

Be aware that in most exercises you will have a tendency to hold your breath too long. This should be avoided because it is dangerous! By not exhaling, you reduce the return of blood to your heart, which in turn reduces the blood flow to the brain. If the brain is deprived of oxygen-rich blood, you will become dizzy and may faint. Holding the breath too long is especially dangerous if you are performing over-head free-weight exercises. If you have high blood pressure, consulting a physician before you begin a weight training program is imperative; once training, you must exhale through the sticking point in each repetition. Learning to exhale at the correct time can be confusing, but the technique sections in this book will tell you when to exhale in each exercise.

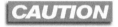 **Do not hold your breath. Exhale through the difficult portion of the exercise.**

SPOTTING

A spotter assists and protects the person lifting from injury. Spotters play a crucial role in making weight training a safe activity.

If you are asked to be a spotter, realize that being inattentive can cause serious injuries (muscle or tendon tears, facial and other bone fractures, broken teeth). Not all exercises require spotters, but the free-weight bench press, back squat, and those involving over-the-head or over-the-face movements do.

Just as you may need to rely on spotters, the person you spot is relying on you. Do not underestimate the significance of your responsibilities as a spotter. Read and adhere to the following guidelines for spotting free-weight exercises and your responsibility to the spotter when you are lifting. Specific instructions for spotting are provided later in this text for the appropriate exercises. Remember: Spotters with poor technique can be injured, too!

1. Remove all loose plates, barbells, and dumbbells from the area to avoid slipping or tripping on them.

2. Learn and practice the spotting techniques and procedures for exercises that involve a spotter.

3. Place your body in a good lifting position in case you have to catch the bar. Keep your knees flexed and your back flat.

4. Effectively communicate with the person you are spotting. For example, before she begins a set, ask her how many reps will be attempted.

5. Use the appropriate grip—a closed grip is a must! Use the proper hand location on the bar if you need to grip it.

6. See that the bar is properly and evenly loaded.

7. Be knowledgeable about potentially dangerous situations associated with each exercise. These are identified throughout this book.

8. Be alert and quick to respond to the needs of the person you are spotting.

9. Know when and how to guide the bar in the desired path.

10. Know when and how much lifting assistance is needed to complete the exercise.

11. As a last resort, assume all of the weight of the bar, but only if the lifter might be injured if you do not take action.

12. Provide the lifter with suggestions about how to improve his technique for each exercise if needed.

As the person performing a weight training exercise, your actions are important to your spotter's safety as well as yours. Following these suggestions will help make training safer for both of you.

1. Tell the spotter the number of reps you intend to complete before you begin the exercise.

2. Be vocal about when you need assistance.

3. Always stay with the bar. That is, once the spotter needs to assist, remember not to let go of the bar or stop trying to complete the exercise. If you do, the spotter must assume the entire weight of the bar and might be injured.

4. Know your strength and technique limitations and select an appropriate load for each set. (This is a common problem for those who are new to training.)

Lifting Fundamentals Drill 1. *Grip Selection and Location*

This drill involves lifting an empty bar or a dowel stick from the floor using the three types of grips in the three grip-width positions described on page 4. When completing this drill, you should position your hands so that the bar is balanced when being pulled to the thighs.

Using an overhand grip (see figure 1.2*a*, page 4), lift the bar to the thighs and then lower it back to the floor using correct lifting techniques. Lift the bar twice more to your thighs, using first the underhand grip (see figure 1.2*b*, page 4) and then the alternated grip (see figure 1.2*c*, page 4).

Now move your hands to the common grip width and use the three different types of grips. Next move your hands to the narrow grip and do the same. Perform all grips with your thumbs around the bar. Check off each correctly performed grip and grip width.

Success Check

- Establish the proper hand spacing.
- Keep your thumbs around the bar.
- Remember the names of the grips.

Score Your Success

Complete three overhand grips with correct technique = 3 points

Complete three underhand grips with correct technique = 3 points

Complete three alternated grips with correct technique = 3 points

Your score ___

Lifting Fundamentals Drill 2. *Preparation Position*

This drill will help you develop a better sense of balance and a greater awareness of proper body positioning.

Without falling forward or allowing either or both heels to rise, squat down into the gorilla position with your hands clasped behind your head. Move into this position 10 times. Performing this drill in front of a mirror is a great way to critique and perfect your technique.

Success Check

- Keep heels on floor and back flat.
- Keep head upright.
- Keep eyes focused straight ahead.

Score Your Success

Give yourself 1 point for each repetition performed with good balance, for a maximum total of 10 points.

Your score ___

Lifting Fundamentals Drill 3. *Floor-to-Thigh*

This drill is designed to help you learn to keep the bar close to your shins, knees, and thighs in order to avoid low back injury when lifting and returning the bar to the floor.

From a standing position, move into the preparatory (gorilla) lifting position. Using the overhand grip, pull the bar to the middle of your thighs. Remember good lifting techniques: head up, back flat, and let the legs do the lifting. Lower the bar to the floor in the same manner. Repeat this drill 10 times. Have a qualified professional check your technique.

Success Check

- Maintain a flat back with your head up.
- Feel the shoulders-back position.
- Keep your hips low.

Score Your Success

Give yourself 1 point for each repetition performed with good lifting technique, based on the evaluation of a qualified professional, for a maximum total of 10 points.

Your score ___

Lifting Fundamentals Drill 4. *Shrug*

Most beginners have a tendency to flex the elbows too soon during what is commonly referred to as the second pull—that is, the pull at the thigh that brings the bar to the shoulders. This drill will help you avoid this common technique flaw.

Using an overhand grip, pick up the bar and hold it at midthigh. With your knees and hips slightly flexed, perform a quick shoulder shrug, then immediately extend your hips and knees while keeping your elbows straight. You may want to think of the movement as jumping with a bar while keeping your elbows straight. After each jump, return the bar to your thighs, not to the floor. Repeat this drill 10 times.

Success Check

• Feel the stretch in the traps.

Score Your Success

Give yourself 1 point for each repetition you complete with straight elbows, for a maximum total of 10 points.

Your score ___

Lifting Fundamentals Drill 5. *Racking the Bar*

This drill will help you develop the timing you need to flex your hips and knees when racking the bar on your shoulders.

Follow the same procedures used in the previous drill, but instead of lowering the bar after the jump, pull it to your shoulders. Work on timing the catch of the bar at your shoulders with the flexing of your hips and knees and with your feet moving to a stance that is somewhat wider than the initial position. Repeat 10 times.

Success Check

• Cushion the catch on the shoulders by flexing the knees.

• Remember to keep your elbows straight until your hips are fully extended.

Score Your Success

Give yourself 1 point for each repetition you successfully complete—hips, knees, and feet properly positioned—for a maximum total of 10 points.

Your score ___

SUCCESS SUMMARY FOR BASICS OF LIFTING AND TRAINING

Weight training should begin with determining if medical clearance is warranted; if so, obtain it before you start a program. Sound training technique requires a proper grip and a stable position from which to lift. You must keep the object being lifted close to your body and use your legs rather than your back. Remember, hips stay low as the legs straighten. This is true regardless of whether you are lifting a barbell or a box off the floor or spotting an exercise. Developing good fundamental techniques will help you avoid injury and work your muscles in ways that produce optimal results.

Before Taking the Next Step

Honestly answer each of the following questions. If you answer yes to all of them, you are ready to move on to step 2.

1. Have you completed the medical clearance checklist (see figure 1.1, page 3) and, if necessary, obtained permission from your doctor to begin a weight training program?
2. Can you identify and perform the three types of grips? Have an experienced lifter observe your technique.
3. Can you identify and perform the four phases of lifting? Have an experienced lifter observe your technique.
4. Do you know how to breathe properly during a repetition?
5. Have you identified an appropriate spotter to assist you in lifts that require one?
6. Have you successfully completed the five drills in this step?

Once you have learned about and practiced fundamental lifting skills and proper breathing and spotting techniques, you are ready to move on to step 2. Step 2 explains a foundational strategy of this book—you will go through five practice activities, called *practice procedures*, to learn how to perform and use the weight training exercises that will make up your new program.

Selecting Exercises and Setting Training Loads

Acquiring the ability to perform weight training exercises correctly creates a sense of accomplishment and pride and enables you to make each training session more satisfying and productive. As you learn the exercises in steps 3 through 9, you will apply the basic techniques you mastered in step 1 and the practice procedures you will learn in this step.

"Practice makes perfect" is the underlying theme for this step. It consists of a series of five practice activities called *practice procedures*. Insight gained from these procedures will help you learn exercises quickly and safely, while increasing your confidence, enjoyment, and weight training success. The procedures are as follows:

1. Choose one exercise for each muscle group.
2. Determine the warm-up and trial loads for each exercise.
3. Practice proper exercise technique.
4. Perform repetitions with the trial load to determine the training load.
5. Make needed adjustments to the training load.

1. CHOOSE ONE EXERCISE

Steps 3 through 8 usually include a choice of one free-weight and two machine exercises that have been selected for those new to weight training because they are easy to learn and perform correctly. All of the exercises in step 9 use free weights. You will choose one exercise for each of the seven muscle groups shown in figure 2.1 and one total-body exercise, then record the exercises selected in the "Exercise" column on the workout chart.

If you are an experienced trainee, consider adding exercises to emphasize muscular size, strength, or endurance in specific areas of the body that are of interest to you. Steps 3 through 8 each include an additional exercise that more experienced trainees may want to include in their programs. These exercises follow the basic exercises in each step and are identified by an asterisk (*). The total body exercises in step 9 are also for lifters with more experience.

For all of the exercises in steps 3 through 9, you should read the technique explanations and then study the illustrations and main technique points. Consider the equipment and spotting requirements of each exercise. Step 10 will explain how to record the exercises you have selected and the loads that you have determined for them on a workout chart.

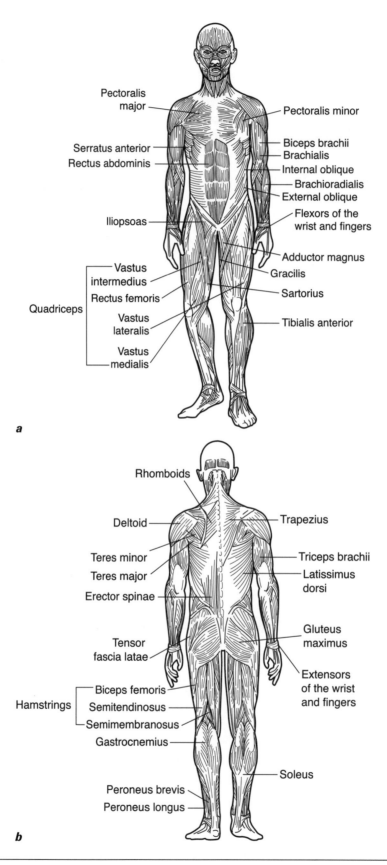

Figure 2.1 Muscle groups: *(a)* anterior, or front, view; *(b)* posterior, or back, view. Exercises for each of these muscle groups are included in the basic program.

2. DETERMINE WARM-UP AND TRIAL LOADS

Using light loads in the early stages of learning weight training exercises enables you to concentrate more on the techniques required and less on how hard to push or pull. Out of enthusiasm or curiosity, you may be tempted to use loads that are too heavy. Selecting loads that are too heavy, even if your technique is perfect, increases the chance of injury. Avoid this temptation!

Provided next are two safe methods for determining warm-up and trial loads. If you are new to weight training, use the first method to determine loads for basic exercises. If you are an experienced trainee, use the second method to determine loads for additional exercises.

Basic Exercises

This practice procedure explains how to use the formulas shown in figure 2.2 to determine the warm-up and trial loads for the basic exercises. If you select one of the first three exercises listed in steps 3 through 8, you will need to identify the coefficient associated with that exercise in figure 2.2. Each step includes exercises and coefficients that are specific to a certain muscle group. Realize that using the coefficients results in *estimated* warm-up and trial loads. Individual differences, combined with the variance in equipment design, make it difficult if not impossible to derive coefficients that are without error. Those presented in this text are starting points for determining appropriate loads. If there is a need to convert pounds to kilograms or kilograms to pounds, refer to the conversion chart on page xxxv.

You will notice that for the first three exercises, the letters FW (for free weight), C (for cam), and M (for multiunit machine—but it can be a single-unit too) identify the type of equipment that is used when performing them.

After you've located the name of the exercise you've selected, write your body weight in the appropriate space and multiply it by the number to the right of it (the coefficient). The use of body weight in determining appropriate loads is based on its relationship to strength. This is the same logic used for creating weight divisions in sports such as wrestling, boxing, and weightlifting.

Calculations of Warm-Up and Trial Loads for Chest Exercises

Body weight	(Exercise)		Coefficient		Trial load	Warm-up load
			Female			
BWT = _120_	(FW–bench press)	×	.35	=	42 lbs. (round off to 40)	20 lbs. (40 ÷ 2)
BWT = _____	(C–pec deck)	×	.14	=	_____	_____
BWT = _____	(M–chest press)	×	.27	=	_____	_____
			Male			
BWT = _____	(FW–bench press)	×	.60	=	_____	_____
BWT = _____	(C–pec deck)	×	.30	=	_____	_____
BWT = _____	(M–chest press)	×	.55	=	_____	_____

BWT = body weight, FW = free weight, C = cam, M = multi- or single-unit machine exercise.

Note: If you are a male who weighs more than 175 lbs. (79 kg), record your body weight as 175 (79). If you are a female who weighs more than 140 lbs. (63.5 kg), record your body weight as 140 (63.5).

Figure 2.2 Calculating warm-up and trial loads for basic exercises.

The coefficient is a number that has been derived from studies of males and females who, for the most part, do not have experience in weight training. When multiplied by your body weight, the coefficient can be used to estimate training loads; using one-half of it provides an appropriate warm-up load.

Note that if you are a male who weighs more than 175 pounds (79 kilograms), you should record your body weight as 175 pounds. If you are a female who weighs more than 140 pounds (64 kilograms), record your body weight as 140 pounds.

To complete this procedure, round off the number to the nearest 5-pound increment or to the closest weight-stack plate. This becomes your trial load. The example seen in figure 2.2 is of a female who weighs 120 pounds and has selected the free-weight bench press from the three chest exercises available. In this example, the rounded-off trial load equals 40 pounds and one-half of that equals a warm-up load of 20 pounds.

Using this method sometimes results in a warm-up load that is lighter than the lightest weight-stack plate on a machine. If this occurs, select the lightest weight plate and recruit an experienced lifter to safely assist (by pushing or pulling) in accomplishing the movement patterns involved in the exercise. The bars available for free-weight exercises may pose the same problems. If so, very light dumbbells, a stripped-down dumbbell bar, a single weight plate, or even a wooden dowel stick (less than a pound in weight) may be used during warm-up sets.

The warm-up load is used in learning the exercise techniques in practice procedure 3, while the trial load is used in practice procedure 4 to determine the training load. Note that we use the term *trial load* because you will be trying it out in practice procedure 4 to see if it is an appropriate load to use later for training. Trial loads that are too heavy or light can be adjusted using practice procedure 5.

*Additional Exercises

If you are an experienced trainee you should consider supplementing the basic workout with one or more of the additional exercises presented in each of steps 3 through 9. If you do, you will need to follow the approach described next to establish training loads for each additional exercise.

Based on your previous experience and awareness of the weight that you can handle, select a weight that will allow you to perform 12 to 15 reps and write it in the "Estimated trial load for 12 to 15 reps" column. Then determine an effective warm-up load by multiplying the trial load by .6 (or use about two-thirds of the trial load if that calculation is easier), and round off the number to the nearest 5-pound increment or to the closest weight-stack plate.

The example seen in figure 2.3 is of an experienced male lifter who wants to add the dumbbell chest fly exercise to his basic program. He estimates that he can lift 35 pounds for 12 to 15 repetitions, which makes his rounded-off warm-up load 20 pounds ($35 \times .6 = 21$, rounded down to 20).

The warm-up load is used in learning the exercise techniques in practice procedure 3, while the trial load is used in practice procedure 4 to determine the training load. Trial loads that are too heavy or light can be adjusted using practice procedure 5.

Calculation of Warm-Up Load for Additional Exercise

Exercise	Estimated trial load for 12-15 reps		Warm-up load
*Dumbbell chest fly	35 lbs.	× .6 =	20 lbs.

Figure 2.3 Example showing how to calculate the warm-up load for an additional exercise, the dumbbell chest fly.

3. PRACTICE PROPER TECHNIQUE

In this practice procedure, you will use warm-up loads while learning each exercise's grip, body positioning, movement pattern, bar velocity, and breathing pattern. Carefully read the information and directions that follow concerning each of these technique considerations and try to apply them during practice procedure 3 in steps 3 through 9.

- **Grip.** As you learned in step 1, a variety of weight training grip styles and grip widths can be used. Learn which type of grip is appropriate and where to place your hands when using that grip in each exercise.

- **Body positioning.** Body positioning refers to the initial posture of the body, not arm or leg movements. Proper positioning in lying down or standing exercises, or on equipment, provides a balanced and stable position from which to pull or push. Improper positioning can reduce the benefits of an exercise or result in serious injury.

- **Movement pattern.** The movement pattern refers to how the arms, legs, and trunk move during the execution of an exercise, and the importance of completing the full range of movement. Performing exercises through the movement ranges and in the patterns shown enables you to get your arms, legs, and trunk more active during each rep and, therefore, better trained. Learning and practicing correct movement patterns and ranges also contribute to safer training sessions.

- **Bar velocity.** Velocity refers to the speed of the barbell, dumbbell, or handle as it moves through the range of motion in an exercise. During this practice procedure, establishing the habit of performing slow, controlled movement patterns is especially important. Try to allow about 2 seconds for the concentric phase (usu-

ally the more difficult, upward movement) and 2 to 4 seconds for the eccentric phase (usually the easier, downward movement) of the exercise. Doing so will avoid the buildup of momentum that is commonly associated with weight training injuries.

- **Breathing pattern.** Trying to remember when to exhale and inhale can be confusing, especially when there are other skills to remember at the same time. As you practice performing exercises with warm-up loads, learn to identify where in each exercise the sticking point occurs and breathe out as described in step 1. Remember that the sticking point in a repetition is the position at which the exercise becomes most difficult. Inhale during the recovery movement phase.

Visualization is an excellent method to help establish correct exercise and spotting techniques. Use all of your senses while visualizing the correct execution of an exercise. Try to find a quiet location in the weight room, or develop the ability, even under noisy conditions, to clearly visualize the proper grip, body positioning, movement pattern, velocity, and breathing for each exercise. Concentrate on feedback from your muscles and joints as you mentally rehearse exercises. This will help you learn how the exercise feels when you are performing it correctly.

You may also want to mimic the correct movement patterns of exercises in front of a mirror, making note of the feedback you sense from muscles, tendons, and joints. Attempt to do this for 1 to 2 minutes immediately before you begin each exercise in practice procedure 2 or 3. Try to find time before each training session to visualize the proper techniques for each exercise until you have mastered them.

4. DETERMINE TRAINING LOAD

The correct load will result in muscular failure on the 12th to 15th rep when maximum effort is given. Simply use the trial load determined in

practice procedure 2 to load the bar or set the machine, and perform as many reps as possible with proper and safe exercise technique. If the number of reps you can complete is 12 to 15, you have found an appropriate training load. Record this number in the training-load column on the workout chart located at the end of step 10 (see page 126). If you performed fewer than 12 or more than 15 reps in any of steps 3 through 9, you have one more practice procedure to complete before moving on to the next exercise.

5. MAKE NEEDED LOAD ADJUSTMENTS

Because individuals differ in physical characteristics and experience and because weight training equipment differs in design, the trial loads may not produce the desired range of 12 to 15 reps. If you performed fewer than 12 reps, the trial load is too heavy. On the other hand, if you performed more than 15 reps, the load is too light.

In this practice procedure, you will use a load-adjustment chart (table 2.1) to make necessary corrections. Once you begin training, you may need to use the chart several times before an accurate training load is determined.

Figure 2.4 shows how the load-adjustment chart is used to make needed adjustments to the trial load for the basic and additional exercises in steps 3 through 9. The example shown is for someone who performed 9 reps with 100 pounds (45 kilograms) in the free-weight bench press exercise. Because only 9 reps (instead of 12 to 15) were performed, the weight was too heavy, and the load needs to be reduced.

Reading across the load adjustment chart, you can see that a 10-pound (4.5-kilogram) reduction is recommended when only 9 reps are performed. The result is a more appropriate training load of 90 pounds (41 kilograms).

Follow these same procedures to adjust the trial load in each exercise, if necessary. Then be sure to record the exercise you selected for the chest at the top of the workout chart, followed by those selected for the back, shoulders, arms (both biceps and triceps), and legs, in that order, as shown in figure 2.5. If you include one of the additional exercises, write it on the workout chart immediately after the basic exercise that you selected (steps 3 through 9).

Table 2.1 Load Adjustments

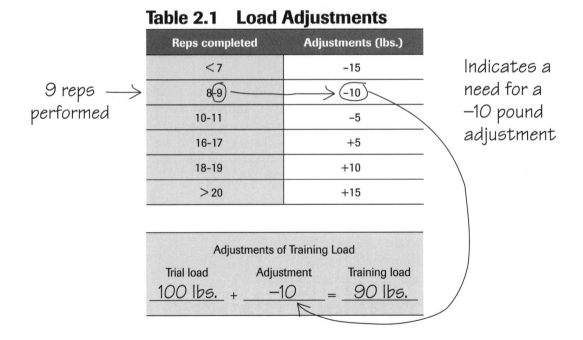

Reps completed	Adjustments (lbs.)
<7	−15
8-9	−10
10-11	−5
16-17	+5
18-19	+10
>20	+15

9 reps performed →

Indicates a need for a −10 pound adjustment

Adjustments of Training Load		
Trial load	Adjustment	Training load
100 lbs. +	−10 =	90 lbs.

Figure 2.4 Example showing how to make a load adjustment. Since this lifter could perform only 9 reps of the free-weight bench press exercise when using a 100-pound training load, he needs to reduce the weight.

Chest Drill 1. Choose One Exercise

After reading about the characteristics and techniques involved in the exercises and the type of equipment required for each, you are ready to put what you have learned to use. Consider the availability of equipment and access to spotters in your situation, then select one of the following exercises to use in your program:

- Free-weight bench press
- Machine pec deck
- Chest press (multi- or single-unit machine)

Write your chest exercise choice on the workout chart in the "Exercise" column (see page 126). If you intend to include the free-weight *dumbbell chest fly exercise, record it on the workout chart immediately after the chest exercise selected above.

Success Check

- Consider availability of equipment.
- Consider need for a spotter and the availability of qualified people.
- Consider time available.
- Choose a chest exercise and record it on the workout chart.

Adjustments of Training Load		
Trial load	Adjustment	Training load
100	−10	90

Weight training workout chart (three days a week)

	Muscle area	Exercise	Load × sets × reps	Set	
1	Total body*			Wt.	
				Reps	
2	Chest	Bench press	90	Wt.	
				Reps	
3	Back	Bent-over row	80	Wt.	
				Reps	
4	Shoulders	Standing press	60	Wt.	
				Reps	
5	Biceps	Biceps curl	75	Wt.	
				Reps	
6	Triceps	Triceps push-down	30	Wt.	
				Reps	
7	Legs	Leg press	165	Wt.	
				Re	

Figure 2.5 Recording exercise selection and training-load information.

Practice Procedures Drill. *Practice Procedure Quiz*

Select the correct answer for each of the following questions. Answers are on page 26.

1. How many primary muscle groups will you choose at least one exercise for?

    a. one

    b. seven

    c. nine

2. What body weight should be multiplied by a coefficient if a male trainee weighs 220 pounds (100 kilograms)?

    a. 140 pounds

    b. 175 pounds

    c. 220 pounds

3. The warm-up load for an additional exercise represents what percent of the estimated trial load?

    a. 40 percent

    b. 50 percent

    c. 60 percent

4. At what point in the movement of an exercise should you inhale?

    a. before each repetition begins

    b. during the sticking point

    c. during the recovery phase

5. In which practice procedure is the trial load used to determine the training load?

    a. practice procedure 3

    b. practice procedure 4

    c. practice procedure 5

6. If you performed 12 to 15 reps with the trial load, should you continue on to practice procedure 5?

    a. yes

    b. no

7. If you performed 17 reps with 100 pounds in practice procedure 4, what should your adjusted training load be?

    a. 105 pounds

    b. 115 pounds

    c. 120 pounds

Score Your Success

Give yourself 1 point for each question you answered correctly, for a maximum total of 7 points.

Your score ____

SUCCESS SUMMARY FOR THE FIVE PRACTICE PROCEDURES

The procedures presented in this step are used in learning the exercises in steps 3 through 9. Begin by selecting one of the exercises shown in each of these steps. Then look up the body-weight coefficient for each exercise and determine the warm-up and trial loads as seen in figure 2.2. If an exercise is new, refer to the instructions and illustrations in steps 3 through 9 to learn the proper technique. Experienced lifters can add any of the additional exercises and determine the warm-up and trial loads as shown in figure 2.3.

If the trial loads are too heavy or too light for the basic or additional exercises, follow the adjustment guidelines in figure 2.4. Using the procedures in the order presented will make learning weight training exercises very easy, especially if you practice visualizing the correct exercise techniques before practice procedures 4 and 5.

Before performing any of the exercises in steps 3 through 9, take time to review and practice the warm-up and cool-down exercises presented in the Fundamentals of Weight Training (see pages xxi-xxxiii). Practicing them will serve as a warm-up and provide an opportunity for you to learn how to perform them correctly. Be sure to start and end each training session with the warm-up and cool-down exercises.

Before Taking the Next Step

Honestly answer each of the following questions. If you answer yes to all of them, you are ready to move on to step 3.

1. Can you list the five practice procedures?
2. Can you determine warm-up and trial loads using sample loads?
3. Can you determine training loads using sample data?
4. Do you understand how to make load adjustments using sample data?
5. Have you completed the practice procedure quiz?

In step 3 you will select the first exercises for your program. This step includes four exercises that can be used to develop the chest, each with specific instructions on how they should be performed, from the grip to the lifting movements involved.

Answer Key

Practice Procedures Drill. *Practice Procedure Quiz*

1. seven

2. 175 pounds

3. 60 percent

4. during the recovery phase

5. practice procedure 4

6. no

7. 105 pounds

Chest Exercises

Some of the most popular exercises in weight training are those that work the chest muscles, or pectorals (pectoralis major and pectoralis minor). When developed properly, these muscles contribute a great deal to an attractive upper body and to success in many recreational and athletic activities.

The bench press, machine pec deck, machine chest press, and the *dumbbell chest fly (an additional exercise) described in this step provide an added benefit because they also work muscles of the front shoulder (anterior deltoid). In addition, the bench press and machine chest press train the back of the upper arms (triceps).

If you have access to free weights, you may select the bench press or the *dumbbell chest fly to develop your chest. If you prefer working with machines, see the sections on the machine pec deck and the machine chest press.

FREE-WEIGHT BENCH PRESS

The free-weight bench press involves the use of a barbell and a bench with uprights, called a *bench press bench*. Begin by sitting on the end of the bench with your back toward the upright supports. Now lie back and position yourself so that your buttocks, shoulders, and head are firmly and squarely on the bench, as shown in figure 3.1a. Your legs should straddle the bench and your feet should be flat on the floor, about shoulder-width apart. This four-point position is important—especially the straddled feet—because it provides stability when you are handling the bar over your chest and face.

From this position, slide toward the upright supports until your eyes are directly below the front edge of the shelf of the uprights. This position helps prevent the bar from hitting the uprights during the upward execution phase but keeps it close enough to be easily placed back on the shelf (racked) after the last repetition. Improper body position on the bench is a common error. Make sure your eyes are below the edge of the shelf and assume the four points of contact.

Misstep

Your body does not have a four point contact with the bench and floor.

Correction

Check to be sure that your head, shoulders, and buttocks are squarely on the bench and both feet are flat on the floor.

While the bar is supported on the uprights, grasp it with an evenly spaced overhand grip, hands about shoulder-width apart or wider. An appropriate grip width on the bar positions the forearms perpendicular to the floor as the bar touches the chest. Keep in mind that a wide grip is preferred because it emphasizes a larger area of the chest than a narrow one does.

Misstep

Your grip is not evenly spaced.

Correction

Evenly space your hands, using the markings on the bar, or have your spotter help you locate a balanced position.

From this position, signal OK to the spotter and push the bar off the uprights to a straight-elbow position with your wrists directly over your elbows. Pause with the bar in the extended-arm position, and then lower it slowly to your chest as shown in figure 3.1*b*. The bar should contact your chest approximately an inch above or below the nipples. A common error is holding the bar too high on the chest. Concentrate on having the bar touch or nearly touch at your nipple area. Inhale as you lower the bar to your chest. Once the bar touches the chest (do not bounce it off your chest), slowly push it straight upward to an extended-elbow position (figure 3.1*c*). If your elbows extend unevenly, visually focus and concentrate on the arm that tends to lag behind. Exhale through the sticking point, which occurs when the bar is about halfway up. Do not allow your wrists to hyperextend (roll back). Concentrate on keeping your wrists in an extended (straight) position.

Misstep

The bar bounces off your chest.

Correction

Control the bar's downward momentum and pause briefly at the chest.

Throughout the exercise keep your head, shoulders, and buttocks in contact with the bench and both feet flat on the floor. Signal the completion of the last repetition by saying OK. Then rack the bar. Be sure to support the bar until it is racked (figure 3.1*d*).

Misstep

Your buttocks lift off the bench, which could cause the bar to move quickly toward your face, possibly causing injury.

Correction

Lighten the load and concentrate on keeping your buttocks in contact with the bench.

Figure 3.1   Free-Weight Bench Press

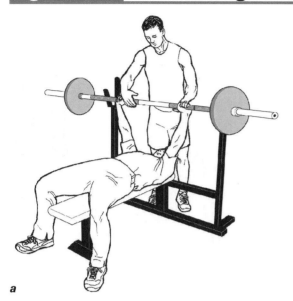

a

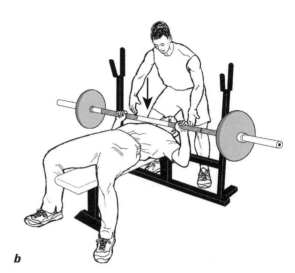

b

Preparation

SPOTTER

1. Use alternated grip, inside partner's hands

2. Place feet hip-width apart, 2 to 6 inches from bench

3. Slightly flex knees

4. Flatten back

5. React to OK command from lifter

6. Assist in lifting bar off supports

7. Guide bar to straight-elbow position

8. Release bar smoothly

LIFTER

1. Take an overhand grip, hands at least shoulder-width apart

2. Create four points of contact: head, shoulders, buttocks on bench; feet on floor

3. Place feet flat on floor as legs straddle bench

4. Focus eyes below edge of shelf

5. Signal OK to spotter

6. Move bar off supports

7. Push to straight-elbow position over chest

8. Keep wrists directly above elbows throughout exercise

Downward Execution

SPOTTER

1. Closely follow downward bar movement with your hands

2. Assist only when necessary

LIFTER

1. Inhale while lowering the bar

2. Keep wrists straight

3. Use slow, controlled movement

4. Touch bar to chest near nipples

5. Pause as bar touches chest

(continued)

Figure 3.1   *(continued)*

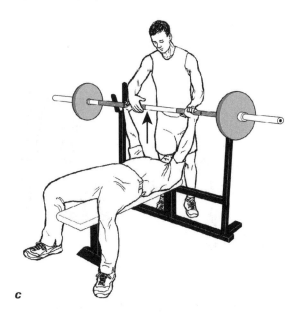

c

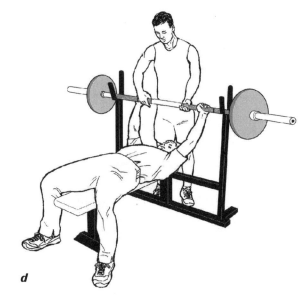

d

Upward Execution

SPOTTER

1. Closely follow bar movement with your hands
2. Watch for uneven arm extension
3. Watch for bar stopping or moving toward lifter's face

LIFTER

1. Push upward with elbows extending evenly
2. Exhale during upward movement
3. Pause at straight-elbow position
4. Continue upward and downward movements until completion of the set
5. Signal OK on the last repetition

Racking the Bar

SPOTTER

1. Grip bar (alternated grip)
2. Keep bar level
3. Guide bar to supports
4. Say OK when bar is racked

LIFTER

1. Keep elbows straight
2. Move bar to supports
3. Support bar until racked

Misstep

When racking, you push the bar into the uprights.

Correction

Visually focus on and maintain control of the bar until it is safely in the rack.

As the spotter, you should stand forward of your partner's head about 2 to 6 inches from the bench and centered between the uprights (figure 3.1a). To assist your partner in moving the bar off the supports (called *handing off*), grip the bar using the alternated grip. Space your hands evenly between your partner's hands. At his OK command, carefully slide the bar off the supports and guide it to a straight-elbow position over his chest. Before releasing the bar, be sure that your partner's elbows are completely straight. Practice making your handoff as smooth as possible. If your handoff is too high, too low, too far forward, or too close to the shelf, it will disturb your partner's stable position on the bench, which may contribute to a poor performance or injury.

Once the downward phase begins, your open hands and eyes should follow under the bar's downward path to the chest (figure 3.1b) and back up to the starting position (figure 3.1c). As the elbows straighten during the last repetition and after your partner has given the OK signal, assist by grasping the bar (figure 3.1d). Be sure that the bar is resting on the shelf of the upright supports before releasing it.

Most errors associated with this exercise are a result of lowering and raising the bar too quickly. Any technique error is made worse as the speed of the movement increases; thus, the first step in correcting errors is to make sure that the bar is moving slowly. Then attempt to make the corrective changes for the errors that apply to you.

MACHINE PEC DECK (SEATED FLY)

If you have access to either a cam or multi- or single-unit machine, you may select the pec deck or the chest press exercise to develop the chest. In this section we cover the machine pec deck.

Assume a sitting position in a pec deck chest machine with your back firmly against the back pad. Adjust the seat until your shoulders are aligned with the overhead cam. Sit erect, looking straight ahead, and place your forearms on the arm pads, with the elbows level with the shoulders. Grip each handle with a closed grip (figure 3.2a).

Misstep

Shoulders are not aligned with the overhead cam.

Correction

Keep your torso in contact with the back pad. If necessary, adjust the seat on the machine.

While in this position, squeeze your forearms together until the pads touch in front of your chest (figure 3.2b). Exhale as your elbows come together. Pause in this position, and then slowly return to the starting position while inhaling (figure 3.2c).

Figure 3.2　　**Machine Pec Deck (Seated Fly)**

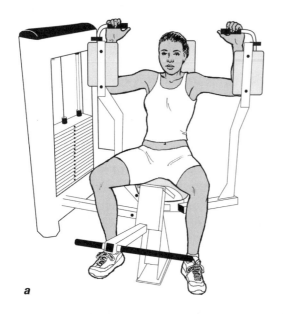

a

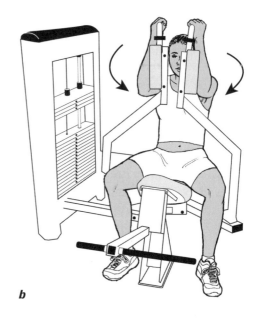

b

PREPARATION

1. Place head, shoulders, and back in contact with back pad
2. Keep shoulders aligned with cam while elbows are together
3. Grip each handle between thumb and index finger
4. Place forearms on arm pads
5. Keep elbows shoulder high

FORWARD EXECUTION

1. Squeeze forearms together; do not pull with hands
2. Keep head and torso on back pad
3. Bring arm pads to front of chest
4. Exhale as elbows come together
5. Pause

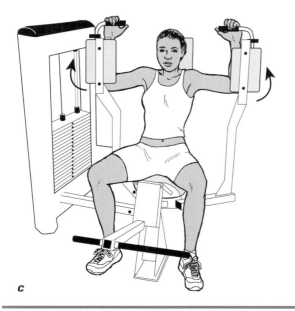

c

BACKWARD EXECUTION

1. Return to starting position
2. Inhale during return to starting position
3. Pause

Misstep

Head and torso lean forward.

Correction

Keep your head and shoulders against the back pad. Lighten the load if necessary.

Misstep

You pull with your hands.

Correction

Think, "Press elbows together."

The machine pec deck is different from the free-weight bench press and the machine chest press in terms of the muscle groups exercised. The triceps are involved in the bench press and chest press but not in the pec deck. The elbow is flexed in a 90-degree angle throughout the pec deck exercise. The free-weight equivalent to the machine pec deck is the dumbbell chest fly (see page 35).

MACHINE CHEST PRESS

Position yourself with head, shoulders, and buttocks in contact with the bench on a multi- or single-unit machine. Put your feet flat on the floor about shoulder-width apart to complete the four points of contact. Grip the bar handles with your hands shoulder-width apart, aligned with your nipples (figure 3.3a).

CAUTION Be sure your head is at least 2 inches (5 centimeters) from the weight stack. If you are too close, the selector key may strike your forehead. Slide toward your feet until the clearance between your head and the weight stack is approximately 2 inches.

From this position, push to a full elbow extension in a slow, controlled manner (figure 3.3b). Exhale through the sticking point. Pause at full extension, then return to the starting position while inhaling (figure 3.3c).

| Figure 3.3 | Chest Press |

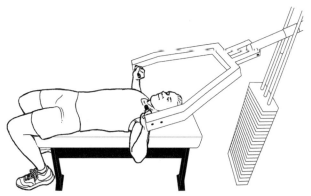

a

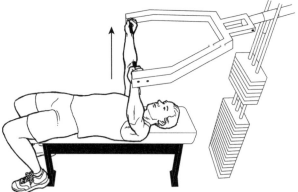

b

PREPARATION

1. Head, shoulders, buttocks stay on bench
2. Feet flat on floor
3. Grip slightly wider than shoulders
4. Grip aligned with nipples

UPWARD EXECUTION

1. Push to full elbow extension
2. Exhale through the sticking point
3. Pause

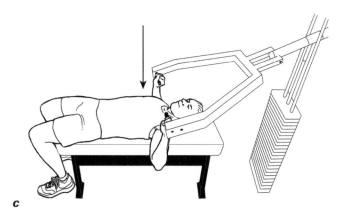

c

DOWNWARD EXECUTION

1. Return to starting position
2. Inhale during downward movement
3. Pause

Misstep

During the downward phase, the weights stop two or more inches above the rest of the weight stack.

Correction

Lower the weight stack until it lightly touches the rest of the stack.

*DUMBBELL CHEST FLY

If you are an experienced lifter who is ready for a more challenging program, consider adding the *dumbbell chest fly exercise. Often this exercise supplements the bench press, machine pec deck, or machine chest press exercise. Being able to move the dumbbells in unison and in an arcing fashion over the chest requires more coordination than the other chest exercises in the basic program. The *dumbbell chest fly involves the same major muscle area as the other exercises—the pectoralis major. This is a pulling exercise.

For the free-weight *dumbbell chest fly, pick up the dumbbells in a neutral grip, palms turned inward. Lie on the bench with head, shoulders, and buttocks in contact with the bench. Place feet flat on the floor, with legs flexed 90 degrees and straddling the bench (figure 3.4a). Flex your arms slightly at the elbows as you hold the dumbbells over your chest.

Inhale as you slowly lower the dumbbells (figure 3.4b). Keep your elbows perpendicular to your torso and slightly flexed. The dumbbells should move in a slight arc, not straight up and down. Lower the dumbbells to chest height, taking care not to twist or arch your body. Keep your head, shoulders, and buttocks in contact with the bench.

Exhale as you return the dumbbells to the starting position (figure 3.4c). Your feet stay flat on the floor and your torso remains in contact with the bench at all times.

Figure 3.4   *Dumbbell Chest Fly

Preparation

SPOTTER

1. Place feet 2 to 6 inches from bench, hip-width apart
2. Keep back flat
3. React to OK command
4. Grasp lifter's wrists or forearms near dumbbells
5. Help lifter move dumbbells into position
6. Guide dumbbells up until lifter's elbows are fully extended
7. Release wrists smoothly

LIFTER

1. Hold dumbbells with neutral grip, palms facing inward
2. Make sure head, shoulders, and buttocks are in contact with bench
3. Flex legs 90 degrees
4. Keep feet flat on floor
5. Slightly flex elbows

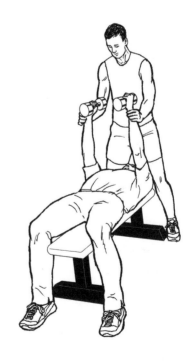

a

(continued)

Figure 3.4 (continued)

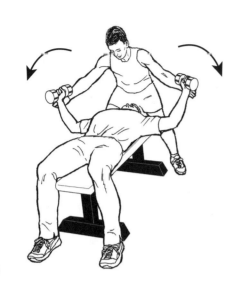

b

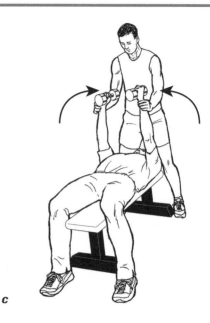

c

Downward Execution

SPOTTER

1. Follow near to (but not touching) lifter's wrists
2. Assist only when necessary

LIFTER

1. Slowly lower dumbbells, keeping elbows perpendicular to torso
2. Lower dumbbells to chest height
3. Keep elbows slightly flexed
4. Do not twist or arch body
5. Inhale while lowering dumbbells

Upward Execution

SPOTTER

1. Follow near to (but not touching) wrists
2. Assist only when necessary

LIFTER

1. Slowly return dumbbells to starting position
2. Keep feet flat on floor
3. Keep head, shoulders, and buttocks on bench
4. Exhale during return

Misstep

You flex your elbows too much.

Correction

Flex the elbows only slightly. Dumbbells should move in a slight arc.

Misstep

Dumbbells are too heavy.

Correction

If you are using dumbbells that are too heavy, you will have to use incorrect technique to compensate, creating the risk of injury. Instead of using improper technique, switch to lighter dumbbells.

Like the free-weight bench press, this exercise also requires a spotter. The spotter should stand forward of the lifter's head about 2 to 6 inches (5 to 15 centimeters) from the bench (figure 3.4a). The spotter either kneels on both knees or positions one knee on the floor with the foot of the other leg forward and flat on the floor. To help the lifter move the dumbbells to the correct starting position, the spotter grasps his wrists or forearms near the dumbbells. At the lifter's OK command, the spotter helps move the dumbbells to a straight-elbow position over the lifter's chest. The spotter releases the dumbbells smoothly after making sure the lifter's elbows are completely straight. When the exercise is performed, the spotter's hands should follow near to (but not touching) the lifter's wrists as he lowers the dumbbells (figure 3.4b) and returns to the starting position (figure 3.4c).

Chest Drill 1. *Choose One Exercise*

After reading about the characteristics and techniques involved in the exercises and the type of equipment required for each, you are ready to put what you have learned to use. Consider the availability of equipment and access to spotters in your situation, then select one of the following exercises to use in your program:

- Free-weight bench press
- Machine pec deck
- Machine chest press (multi- or single-unit machine)

Write your chest exercise choice on the workout chart in the "Exercise" column (see page 126). If you intend to include the free-weight *dumbbell chest fly exercise, record it on the workout chart immediately after the chest exercise selected above.

Success Check

- Consider availability of equipment.
- Consider need for a spotter and the availability of qualified people.
- Consider time available.
- Choose a chest exercise and record it on the workout chart.

Chest Drill 2. *Warm-Up and Trial Loads for Basic Exercises*

This practice procedure will ultimately answer the question "How much weight or load should I use?" Using the coefficient associated with the chest exercise you selected and the formula shown in figure 3.5, determine the trial load. (See step 2, pages 18-20, for more information on using this formula.) Round your results to the nearest 5-pound (2.25-kilogram) increment or to the closest weight-stack plate. Be sure to use the coefficient assigned to the exercise you selected. Use one-half of the amount determined for the trial load for your warm-up load in the exercise. These loads will be used in drills 4 and 5.

Success Check

- Determine your trial load by multiplying your body weight by the correct coefficient.
- Determine your warm-up load by dividing your trial load by two.
- Round off your trial and warm-up loads to the nearest weight stack or bar weight.
- Write down your warm-up and trial loads.

Calculations of Warm-Up and Trial Loads for Chest Exercises

Body weight	(Exercise)		Coefficient		Trial load	Warm-up load
			Female			
BWT = _____	(FW–bench press)	×	.35	=	_____	_____
BWT = _____	(C–pec deck)	×	.14	=	_____	_____
BWT = _____	(M–chest press)	×	.27	=	_____	_____
			Male			
BWT = _____	(FW–bench press)	×	.60	=	_____	_____
BWT = _____	(C–pec deck)	×	.30	=	_____	_____
BWT = _____	(M–chest press)	×	.55	=	_____	_____

BWT = body weight, FW = free weight, C = cam, M = multi- or single-unit machine exercise.

Note: If you are a male who weighs more than 175 lbs. (79 kg), record your body weight as 175 (79). If you are a female who weighs more than 140 lbs. (63.5 kg), record your body weight as 140 (63.5).

Figure 3.5 Warm-up and trial load determination for basic chest exercises.

Chest Drill 3. *Determine Trial Load for *Dumbbell Chest Fly*

If you are an experienced lifter who has decided to add the *dumbbell chest fly, follow the directions to determine your trial load. (See step 2, pages 18-20, for more information.)

Based on your previous experience and knowledge of the weight you can lift, select a weight that will allow you to perform 12 to 15 reps. Calculate the warm-up load by multiplying the trial load by .6, and round off the number to the nearest 5-pound increment (figure 3.6). These loads will be used in drill 4.

Success Check

- Select a weight that will allow 12 to 15 reps.
- Determine the warm-up load by multiplying the trial load by .6.
- Round off the warm-up load to the nearest 5-pound increment.
- Write down your warm-up and trial loads.

Calculation of Warm-Up Load for Additional Exercise

Exercise	Estimated trial load for 12-15 reps	Warm-up load
*Dumbbell chest fly	_____ × .6 =	_____

Figure 3.6 Formula for determining the warm-up load for the *dumbbell chest fly.

Chest Drill 4. *Practice Proper Technique*

In this procedure, you are to perform 15 reps with the warm-up load determined in drill 2 (free-weight bench press, machine pec deck, or machine chest press) or drill 3 (*dumbbell chest fly). If you are an experienced lifter who has decided to add the *dumbbell chest fly, practice it last.

Review the illustrations and instructions for the exercise, focusing on proper grip and body positioning. Visualize the movement pattern through the full range of motion. Inhale when you are ready to execute the exercise, then perform the movement with a slow, controlled velocity, remembering to exhale through the sticking point. Ask a qualified lifter to observe and assess your technique.

If you selected the free-weight bench press or the *dumbbell chest fly, you need a spotter. You also need to practice spotting these exercises. Identify a spotter with whom you will take turns completing the drill.

Instead of performing 15 reps in a continuous manner, rack the bar (free-weight bench press) or return the dumbbells to the floor (*dumbbell chest fly) after each repetition to practice the bench press handoff or the *dumbbell chest fly wrist grasp at the beginning of each repetition. Alternate responsibilities so that you and your partner both have a chance to develop the techniques that are required in performing and spotting these exercises. Ask a qualified person to observe and assess your performance in the basic techniques.

Success Check

- For the free-weight bench press, all handoffs and rackings are correctly performed.
- For the *dumbbell chest fly, all wrist grasps are correctly performed.
- For all exercises, movement pattern, velocity, and breathing are correct.

Chest Drill 5. *Determine Training Load*

This practice procedure will help you determine an appropriate training load designed to produce 12 to 15 reps. For basic exercises, perform as many reps as possible with the calculated trial load from drill 2. Make sure that the reps are correctly executed.

If you executed 12 to 15 reps with the trial load, then your trial load is your training load. Record this weight as your training load for this

exercise on the workout chart (see page 126). If you did not perform 12 to 15 reps, go to drill 6 to make adjustments to the load.

Success Check

- Check for correct load.
- Maintain proper and safe technique during each rep.

Chest Drill 6. *Make Needed Load Adjustments*

If you performed fewer than 12 reps with your trial load, the load is too heavy and you need to lighten it. On the other hand, if you performed more than 15 reps, the trial load is too light and you need to increase it. Use table 3.1 to determine the adjustment you need to make. Figure 3.7 shows the formula for making load adjustments.

Success Check

- Check correct use of the load-adjustment chart (table 3.1).
- Record your training load on the workout chart (see page 126).

Table 3.1 Load Adjustments

Reps completed	Adjustments (lbs.)
< 7	−15
8-9	−10
10-11	−5
16-17	+5
18-19	+10
> 20	+15

Adjustments of Training Load

Trial load	Adjustment	Training load
_____ +	_____ =	_____

Figure 3.7 Making adjustments to the training load for chest exercises.

SUCCESS SUMMARY FOR CHEST EXERCISES

This step involved selecting one chest exercise for which you have the needed equipment, and perhaps one more if you have already been training. Using a proper grip; the correct body position, movement, and breathing patterns; and accurate warm-up and training loads will ensure a positive outcome.

Once you have determined your training load and recorded it on your workout chart, you are ready to move on to step 4. In this step you will select exercises that develop the back muscles. It includes four exercises, each with specific instructions on how they should be performed, from the grip to the lifting movements involved.

Before Taking the Next Step

Honestly answer each of the following questions. If you answer yes to all of the questions relevant to your level and exercise selection, you are ready to move on to step 4.

1. Have you selected a basic chest exercise? If you are an advanced lifter, do you want to add the *dumbbell chest fly?

2. Have you recorded your exercise selection (or selections) on the workout chart?

3. Have you determined a warm-up and training load for the exercise(s) you selected?

4. Have you recorded the warm-up and training loads on the workout chart?

5. Have you learned the proper technique for performing the exercise(s) you selected?

6. If the exercise requires a spotter, have you identified a qualified person? Have you learned the proper spotting techniques?

Back Exercises

The bent-over row using free weights, the machine row that uses a cam machine, and the seated row and *lat pull-down (both of which require a multi- or single-unit machine) are excellent exercises to develop the upper back. These muscles—the rhomboids, trapezius, latissimus dorsi, and teres major—work in opposition to those of the chest. These exercises also develop the back of the shoulder (posterior deltoid, infraspinatus, teres minor), the front of the upper arm (biceps brachii), and the back of the forearm (brachioradialis). Back exercises should be performed as often as chest exercises to keep the anterior and posterior upper-body musculature in balance.

If you have access to free weights, select the bent-over row to develop your back. If you have access to either a cam or multi- or single-unit machine, you may select the machine row, the seated row, or the *lat pull-down exercise.

BENT-OVER ROW

Begin with your feet shoulder-width apart and your shoulders slightly higher—10 to 30 degrees—than your hips (figure 4.1a). Your back should be flat, abdominal muscles contracted, elbows straight, knees slightly flexed, and eyes looking forward. Grasp the bar in a palms-down overhand grip with thumbs around the bar. Your hands should be evenly spaced 4 to 6 inches (10 to 15 centimeters) wider than shoulder-width.

Pull the bar upward in a straight line (figure 4.1b). Exhale as the bar nears your chest during the upward movement. Pull in a slow, controlled manner until the bar touches your chest near the nipples (or, for women, just below your breasts). Your torso should remain straight and rigid throughout the exercise, with no bouncing or jerking.

Misstep

The bar does not touch your chest.

Correction

Reduce the weight on the bar and concentrate on touching your chest with the bar.

When the bar touches your chest, pause momentarily before beginning the downward movement (figure 4.1*c*). Inhale during the downward movement. Slowly lower the bar in a straight line to the starting position without letting the weight touch the floor or bounce at the bottom.

Be sure to keep your knees slightly flexed during the upward and downward movements to avoid putting undue stress on your low back.

Misstep

Your upper back is rounded.

Correction

Lift your head, slightly arch your back, and look straight forward.

Misstep

Your knees are locked.

Correction

Flex your knees slightly to reduce stress on your low back.

Figure 4.1   Bent-Over Row (Free Weight)

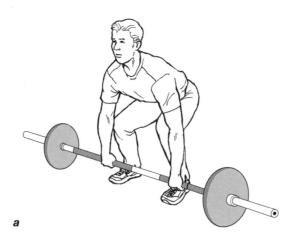

a

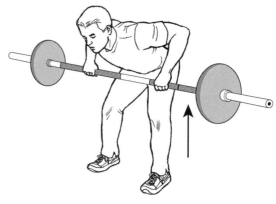

b

PREPARATION

1. Use overhand grip, hands at least shoulder-width apart
2. Keep shoulders higher than hips
3. Keep low back flat
4. Keep elbows straight
5. Slightly flex knees
6. Hold head up, face forward

RAISE THE BAR

1. Slowly pull bar straight up
2. Pause momentarily as bar touches chest
3. Touch chest near nipples (below breasts for women)
4. Keep torso rigid
5. Exhale as bar nears chest

LOWER THE BAR

1. Slowly lower bar straight down

2. Do not bounce or jerk weight at bottom of movement

3. Do not allow weight to touch floor

4. Inhale during downward movement

5. Continue upward and downward movements until set is complete

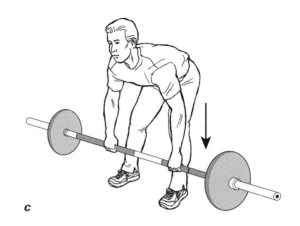

c

Misstep

Your upper torso is not stable and moves up and down.

Correction

Use a mirror to watch and maintain the proper position, or have someone place a hand on your upper back.

Misstep

On the upward movement, you quickly drop your chest to make contact with the bar.

Correction

If you cannot pull the bar to your chest with strict form, you should lighten the weight.

Special caution: Although the bent-over row is considered to be one of the best exercises for the upper back, it is also frequently performed with bad technique or modified more than usual. Do not be tempted to use heavier weights, thinking that it will increase your strength faster. Do not try to impress your friends and other people in the weight room. Attempting to lift too much weight leads to bad technique and possible injury. One of the easiest mistakes you can make is to use a heavier weight than you can handle. Another is to pull upward, simultaneously lifting with your legs and low back, and then quickly dropping your chest to make contact with the bar. Dropping your chest quickly puts great stress on the low back, increases your risk of injury, and does little to improve the strength of the upper back.

A common modification for the bent-over row is to place the forehead on something to brace the back so that the neck supports some of the weight. There are arguments for and against this practice, but we are against using a head support. First, if you need to use this technique you are probably attempting to lift too much weight and might injure the vertebrae in your neck. Second, if the proper stance is taken and good technique followed, the extra support is not needed. Third, if your low back cannot support this movement without additional support, then you should concentrate on strengthening that area.

Most errors associated with the bent-over row derive from using too much weight and not maintaining the proper body position. When too much weight is used, the back muscles cannot pull the bar all the way to the chest, which reduces the extent to which those muscles can be worked and developed. You will tend to jerk the bar, using momentum to get it to the chest, then let it free-fall back to the starting position. Avoiding the use of too-heavy loads will enable you to work the back muscles more effectively because you will be able to pull the bar all the way to your chest. Establishing and maintaining the proper body position is also important. A correct shoulder-to-back position places the back muscles in an ideal alignment for strengthening and reduces the likelihood of injury to the low back.

MACHINE ROW

Equipment designs for the machine row vary. Your exercise facility may not have the type of machine shown in figure 4.2. If not, ask for assistance and learn the proper technique from a qualified instructor.

Assume a sitting position in the cam rowing machine with your back toward the weight stack. Sit erect, look straight ahead, and place your upper arms between the pads with your forearms crossed (figure 4.2a).

While maintaining the preparatory body position, pull your arms as far back as possible, similar to a rowing movement (figure 4.2b). Exhale. Pause and then return slowly to the starting position while inhaling (figure 4.2c). Keep your forearms parallel to the floor at all times.

| Figure 4.2 | Machine Row (Cam Machine) |

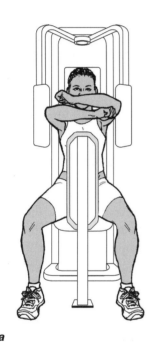 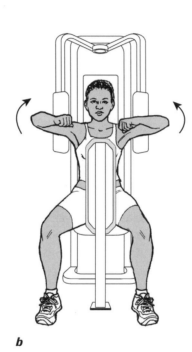 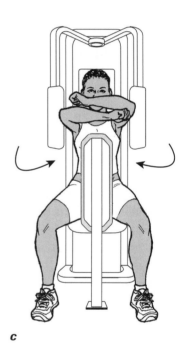

a

PREPARATION

1. Sit with back toward weight stack
2. Place upper arms between pads
3. Cross forearms

b

ROW BACK

1. Pull arms in a rowing movement as far back as possible
2. Keep forearms parallel to floor at all times
3. Exhale while pulling
4. Pause

c

RETURN

1. Slowly return to starting position
2. Inhale

Misstep

You do not complete the full range of motion.

Correction

Bring your elbows back until they form a straight line with each other.

Misstep

Your forearms are not parallel to the floor.

Correction

Keep your palms facing the floor at all times.

SEATED ROW

At the low-pulley station, get into a seated position with your knees slightly flexed (figure 4.3a). Keep your torso erect, with your low back and abdominal muscles contracted. Grip the handles with palms facing inward.

Misstep

Your knees are straight rather than flexed slightly.

Correction

Make sure your knees are slightly flexed to decrease pressure on your low back.

Misstep

Your torso is rounded rather than erect.

Correction

Keep your torso erect by contracting your abdominal and low back muscles.

Maintain this position as you pull the bar slowly and smoothly to your chest (figure 4.3b). Exhale as the bar nears your chest. Pause, then return to the starting position while inhaling (figure 4.3c). Your upper torso should not move back and forth; keep it rigid and, if necessary, lighten the weight.

| Figure 4.3 | Seated Row (Multi- or Single-Unit Machine) |

PREPARATION

1. Assume a seated position
2. Slightly flex knees
3. Keep upper torso erect
4. Keep low back flat
5. Grip handle with palms turned inward

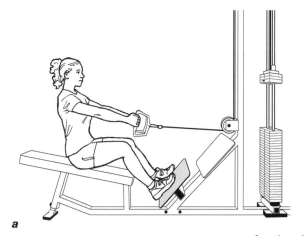

a

(continued)

Figure 4.3 *(continued)*

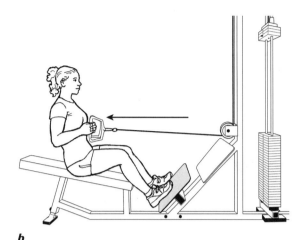

b

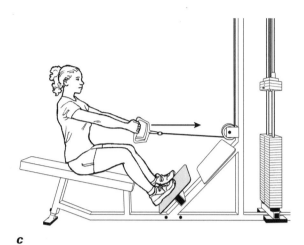

c

PULL

1. Pull handle slowly and smoothly to chest
2. Do not use torso movement to pull weight
3. Exhale as bar nears chest
4. Pause

RETURN

1. Return to starting position
2. Inhale

Misstep

You allow the weight plate to fall quickly onto the stack.

Correction

Pause at your chest, then slowly return the bar to the starting position. Maintain control of the weight all the way through the exercise.

The most common error committed during the seated row exercise is to allow the upper body to move forward and backward instead of remaining erect throughout the exercise. When this happens, the low back muscles become involved in pulling. This compromises the benefit to the upper back muscles for which this exercise was designed.

*LAT PULL-DOWN

A common supplementary exercise for the upper back is the *lat pull-down. It is similar to the pull-up but it is performed in a multi- or single-unit machine.

This pulling exercise develops the upper back (latissimus dorsi, rhomboids, trapezius) and involves some anterior upper-arm (biceps) muscles. It can be performed sitting in a machine (as shown in figure 4.4) or kneeling on the floor.

Begin by assuming an upright, seated position facing the weight stack with your legs straddling the thigh support post and your feet flat on the floor. Take the bar in an overhand grip, with hands slightly wider than shoulder-width (figure 4.4a). Slightly tilt the torso back and extend the arms.

Smoothly pull the bar straight down in front of your face and past your chin (figure 4.4b). Keep your elbows out and away from your body. Touch your upper chest with the bar. Exhale as the bar touches your chest.

To return the bar to the starting position, slowly extend the arms upward, raising the bar (figure 4.4c). Control the weight; do not allow the weight plate to hit the stack. Inhale as you fully extend your arms.

Figure 4.4 *Lat Pull-Down (Multi- or Single-Unit Machine)

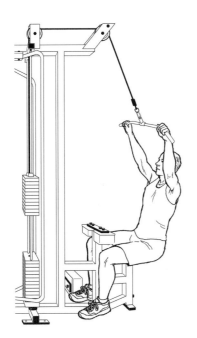

a

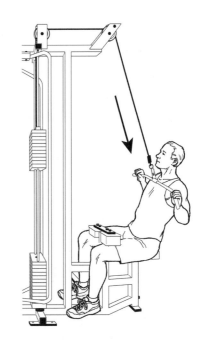

b

PREPARATION

1. Use an overhand grip
2. Place hands slightly farther than shoulder-width apart
3. Assume kneeling or seated position
4. Tilt torso back slightly
5. Extend arms

PULL

1. Pull bar straight down in front of face
2. Pull smoothly
3. Keep elbows out and away from body
4. Pull bar past chin until it touches upper chest
5. Exhale as bar touches chest

(continued)

Figure 4.4 *(continued)*

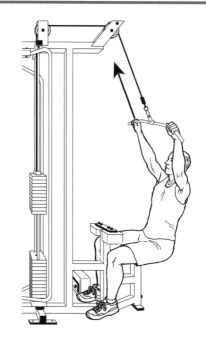

RETURN

1. Slowly extend arms upward
2. Do not allow weight plate to hit weight stack
3. Fully extend arms
4. Inhale while extending arms

c

Misstep

You use your torso to complete the movement.

Correction

Keep the torso erect. Use your back, arm, and shoulder muscles.

Misstep

You allow the weight plate to drop quickly and hit the stack.

Correction

Pause when the bar touches your chest. Control the weight. Slowly return the bar to the starting position. Do not let the weight plate hit the stack.

Back Drill 1.   *Choose One Exercise*

After reading about the characteristics and techniques of the exercises and the type of equipment required for each, you are ready to put what you have learned to use. Consider the availability of equipment in your situation, then select one of the following exercises to use in your program:

- Bent-over row (free weight)
- Machine row (cam machine)
- Seated row (multi- or single-unit machine)

Write your back exercise choice on the workout chart in the "Exercise" column (see page 126). If you intend to include the machine *lat pull-down exercise, record it on the workout chart immediately after the previously selected back exercise.

Success Check

- Consider availability of equipment.
- Consider time available.
- Choose a back exercise and record it on the workout chart.

Back Drill 2. *Warm-Up and Trial Loads for Basic Exercises*

This practice procedure will answer the question "How much weight or load should I use?" Using the coefficient associated with the back exercise you selected and the formula shown in figure 4.5, determine the trial load. (See step 2, pages 18-20, for more information on using this formula.) Round your results to the nearest 5-pound increment or to the closest weight-stack plate. Be sure to use the coefficient assigned to the exercise you selected. Use one-half of the amount determined for the trial load for your warm-up load in the exercise. These loads will be used in drills 4 and 5.

Success Check

- Determine your trial load by multiplying your body weight by the correct coefficient.
- Determine your warm-up load by dividing your trial load by two.
- Round off your trial and warm-up loads to the nearest 5-pound increment or to the closest weight-stack plate.
- Write down your warm-up and trial loads.

Calculations of Warm-Up and Trial Loads for Back Exercises

Body weight	(Exercise)		Coefficient		Trial load	Warm-up load
		Female				
BWT = _____	(FW–bent-over row)	×	.35	=	_____	_____
BWT = _____	(C–machine row)	×	.20	=	_____	_____
BWT = _____	(M–seated row)	×	.25	=	_____	_____
		Male				
BWT = _____	(FW–bent-over row)	×	.45	=	_____	_____
BWT = _____	(C–machine row)	×	.40	=	_____	_____
BWT = _____	(M–seated row)	×	.45	=	_____	_____

BWT = body weight, FW = free weight, C = cam, M = multi- or single-unit machine exercise.

Note: If you are a male who weighs more than 175 lbs. (79 kg), record your body weight as 175 (79). If you are a female who weighs more than 140 lbs. (63.5 kg), record your body weight as 140 (63.5).

Figure 4.5 Trial load determination for basic back exercises.

Back Drill 3. *Determine Trial Load for *Lat Pull-Down*

If you are an experienced lifter who has decided to add the *lat pull-down, follow the directions to determine the trial load. (See step 2, pages 18-20, for more information.)

Based on your previous experience and knowledge of the weight that you can lift, select a weight that will allow you to perform 12 to 15 reps. Calculate the warm-up load by multiplying the trial load by .6, and round off the number to the closest weight-stack plate (figure 4.6). These loads will be used in drill 4.

Calculation of Warm-Up Load for Additional Exercise

Exercise	Estimated trial load for 12-15 reps	Warm-up load
*Lat pull-down	_____ × .6 =	_____

Figure 4.6 Formula for determining the warm-up load for the lat pull-down.

Success Check

- Select a weight that will allow 12 to 15 reps.
- Determine the warm-up load by multiplying the trial load by .6.
- Round off the warm-up load to the closest weight-stack plate.
- Write down your warm-up and trial loads.

Back Drill 4.   *Practice Proper Technique*

In this procedure, you are to perform 15 reps with the warm-up load determined in drill 2 (bent-over row, machine row, or seated row) or drill 3 (*lat pull-down). If you are an experienced lifter who has decided to add the *lat pull-down, practice it last.

Review the illustrations and instructions for the exercise, focusing on proper grip and body positioning. Visualize the movement pattern through the full range of motion. Inhale when you are ready to execute the exercise, then perform the movement with a slow, controlled velocity, remembering to exhale through the sticking point. Ask a qualified lifter to observe and assess your technique.

Success Check

- Check movement pattern.
- Check velocity.
- Check breathing.

Back Drill 5.   *Determine Training Load*

This practice procedure will help you determine an appropriate training load designed to produce 12 to 15 reps. For basic exercises, perform as many reps as possible with the calculated trial load from drill 2. Make sure that you execute the reps correctly. If you are doing the free-weight bent-over row, also check that your hips are lower than your back and that the bar touches at or near the nipples.

If you executed 12 to 15 reps with the trial load, then your trial load is your training load.

Record this weight as your training load for this exercise in the workout chart (see page 126). If you did not perform 12 to 15 reps, go to drill 6 to make adjustments to the load.

Success Check

- Check for correct load.
- Maintain proper and safe technique during each rep.

Back Drill 6.   *Make Needed Load Adjustments*

If you performed fewer than 12 reps with your trial load, the load is too heavy and you need to lighten it. On the other hand, if you performed more than 15 reps, the trial load is too light and you need to increase it. Use table 4.1 to determine the adjustment you need to make. Figure 4.7 shows the formula for making load adjustments.

Success Check

- Check correct use of load-adjustment chart (table 4.1).
- Record your training load on the workout chart (see page 126).

Table 4.1   Load Adjustments

Reps completed	Adjustments (lbs.)
<7	−15
8-9	−10
10-11	−5
16-17	+5
18-19	+10
>20	+15

Adjustments of Training Load

Trial load	Adjustment	Training load
_____ +	_____ =	_____

Figure 4.7 Making adjustments to the training load for back exercises.

SUCCESS SUMMARY FOR BACK EXERCISES

This step involved selecting one back exercise for which you have the needed equipment, and perhaps one more if you have already been training. Using a proper grip; the correct body position, movement, and breathing patterns; and accurate warm-up and training loads will ensure a positive outcome.

Before Taking the Next Step

Honestly answer each of the following questions. If you answer yes to all of the questions relevant to your level and exercise selection, you are ready to move on to step 5.

1. Have you selected a basic back exercise? If you are an advanced lifter, do you want to add the *lat pull-down?
2. Have you recorded your exercise selection (or selections) on the workout chart?
3. Have you determined a warm-up and training load for the exercise(s) you selected?
4. Have you recorded the warm-up and training loads on the workout chart?
5. Have you learned the proper technique for performing the exercise(s) you selected?

Once you have determined your training load and recorded it on your workout chart, you are ready to move on to step 5. In step 5 you will select exercises that will develop the shoulder muscles, including the standing press; seated press; shoulder press (using free weights or a cam or pivot machine) and the *upright row.

Shoulder Exercises

Overhead pressing exercises using free weights, a pulley or pivot machine, or a cam machine are excellent for developing the front, middle, and posterior sections of the shoulder (anterior, middle, and posterior heads of the deltoid). They also develop the back of the upper arm (triceps). These exercises contribute to shoulder-joint stabilization and muscle padding for protection, as well as balancing muscular development of the chest and upper back.

The free-weight standing press, also called the military press, is generally considered to be the best shoulder exercise, although the free-weight *upright row is a good alternative because it does not involve (and therefore fatigue) the triceps.

If you have access to free weights, you may select the standing press or the *upright row to develop your shoulders. If you have access to either a multi- or single-unit or a cam machine, you may select the seated press exercise or shoulder press exercise to develop your shoulders. They involve nearly the same movements but are performed with different types of machines.

STANDING PRESS

To prepare for this exercise, place the bar on a squat rack or set of supports at shoulder height. If racks or supports are not available, you must lift the bar from the floor, utilizing the techniques presented in step 1.

Grasp the bar in an overhand grip, with your hands equidistant from the center of the bar and slightly more than shoulder-width apart. Hold your wrists firmly in a slightly extended position with elbows under the bar. The bar should be resting on your shoulders, clavicles (collarbones), and hands (figure 5.1a).

Misstep

Your grip is too wide.

Correction

Evenly space your hands, using the markings on the bar for reference.

Push the bar upward in a straight line above your shoulders at a slow to moderate speed, until your elbows are extended (figure 5.1*b*). You will need to move your head slightly backward as the bar moves off and returns to the

shoulders. Otherwise, maintain your head in an upright position throughout this exercise. Avoid leaning back or hyperextending the spine (exaggerating the low back curvature) during the press.

Misstep

You start the bar upward with a knee kick (flexion, then a quick extension).

Correction

Start with your knees in a fully extended position and keep them that way throughout the upward and downward movements of the bar.

Pause momentarily at the top, then lower the bar slowly to the ready position (figure 5.1*c*). Do not bounce the bar on your upper chest. Inhale as you lower the bar and exhale as it passes through the sticking point on ascent. After the last repetition, rack the bar as shown in figure 5.1*d*. If you must lower the bar to the floor after completing the exercise,

use the shoulder-to-floor lowering techniques presented in step 1.

CAUTION Be careful not to hold your breath through the sticking point; doing so could cause you to pass out. Exhale as the bar reaches the sticking point.

Figure 5.1 Standing Press (Free Weight)

Preparation

SPOTTER

1. Stand directly behind partner
2. Stand as close as possible without touching
3. Watch the bar
4. Keep feet shoulder-width apart

LIFTER

1. Use an overhand grip, hands evenly spaced, shoulder-width or slightly wider
2. Hold head upright, facing forward
3. Position elbows under bar, wrists extended
4. Hold bar in hands, resting it on shoulders and clavicles

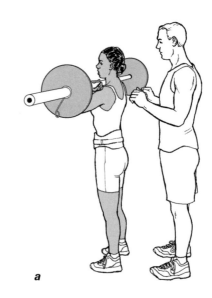

a

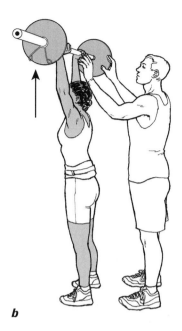

b

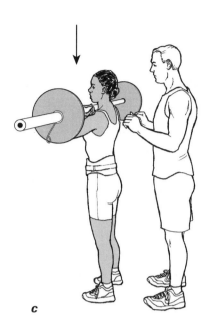

c

Upward Execution

SPOTTER

1. Keep hands close to bar, tracking upward movement
2. Assist only if necessary
3. Caution partner not to lean back or hold breath

LIFTER

1. Push bar straight up
2. Keep back flat and erect
3. Exhale through sticking point
4. Pause at top of movement

Downward Execution

SPOTTER

1. Keep hands close to bar, tracking downward movement
2. Watch for excessive bar speed
3. Caution partner not to bounce bar off upper chest

LIFTER

1. Lower bar slowly
2. Do not bounce bar off upper chest
3. Inhale on descent

Rack the Bar

SPOTTER

1. Walk with partner until bar is racked
2. Tell partner when bar is safely racked

LIFTER

1. Walk forward until bar contacts rack
2. Bend knees to place bar in rack
3. Never lean forward to rack bar

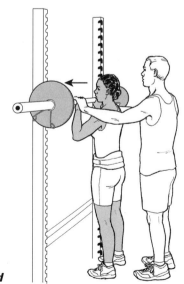

d

Misstep

Your eyes are closed during the exercise.

Correction

Focus on an object straight ahead, especially when you reach the sticking point.

Misstep

Your arms extend unevenly.

Correction

Keep both arms moving in unison upward by visually focusing and concentrating on the arm that lags behind.

As the spotter, you should stand directly behind your partner as close as you can without causing contact (figure 5.1a). With outstretched arms and your open hands under (but not touching) the bar, follow it as it moves up and down (figures 5.1b and c). Once your partner has given the OK signal after the last repetition, assist by grasping the bar (figure 5.1d) and help return it to the rack supports before releasing it.

Of the errors commonly seen in the standing press, leaning back too far is the most common. This typically occurs at the bar's sticking point. It should be avoided because it places a lot of stress on the low back. Think, "Torso, head, and bar form a straight line."

SEATED PRESS

Assume an erect sitting position on the stool of the multi- or single-unit weight machine so that the fronts of your shoulders are directly below the handles (figure 5.2a). Take a palms-forward grip with hands approximately shoulder-width apart.

Push the handles up until your elbows extend completely (figure 5.2b). Keep your shoulders directly under the handles throughout the exercise. Keep your low back flat by statically contracting those muscles and your abdominal muscles. Exhale as your elbows near the fully extended (sticking point) position. Pause when your elbows are fully extended, then slowly return to the starting position (figure 5.2c).

The most common errors made during the seated press are hyperextending (excessively arching) the low back and failing to lower the handles to shoulder level. Hyperextending the low back applies a great deal of stress to it. Keep it flat by contracting your abdominal and low back muscles. Think, "Head, torso, and buttocks form a straight line."

Failing to lower the handles to the starting position reduces the range through which the shoulder muscles are exercised, thus minimizing their development. Try to lower the handles enough so that the weight plate lightly touches (not bangs) the weight stack. To keep the weight plates from banging against each other, control the handles' downward momentum and pause at shoulder level before pushing upward for the next rep.

Figure 5.2   Seated Press (Multi- or Single-Unit Machine)

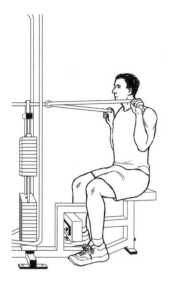

a

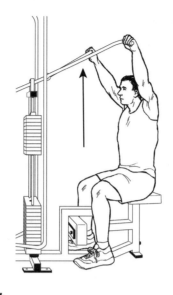

b

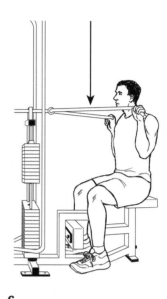

c

PREPARATION

1. Sit on stool or seat so that fronts of shoulders are directly below handles

2. Grip handles with palms forward

3. Place hands approximately shoulder-width apart

4. Keep shoulders directly under handles

5. Keep low back flat

UPWARD EXECUTION

1. Push up to complete extension

2. Exhale during upward movement

3. Pause

RETURN

1. Return to starting position

2. Inhale on downward movement

Misstep

You hold your breath.

Correction

Begin to exhale when the handles reach the sticking point.

SHOULDER PRESS

Position yourself on the seat of the cam machine with your back against the pad and your shoulders aligned under the handles. Grasp the handles with a palms-inward grip (figure 5.3a).

From this position, push to full elbow extension in a slow, controlled manner (figure 5.3b). Exhale when passing through the sticking point. Pause at full extension, then return to the starting position while inhaling (figure 5.3c).

| Figure 5.3 | Shoulder Press (Cam Machine) |

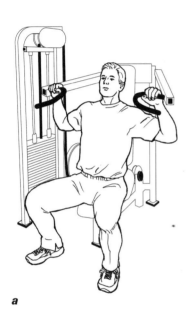

a

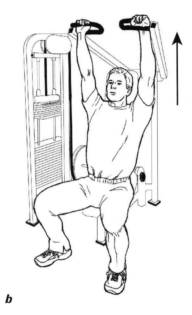

b

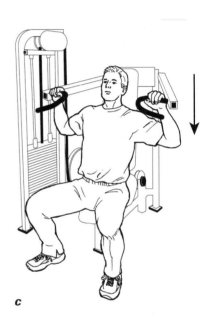

c

PREPARATION

1. Assume a seated position against pad
2. Grip the handles with palms facing forward

LIFT

1. Push up to complete extension
2. Keep elbows directly under wrists
3. Exhale through sticking point of upward movement
4. Pause at top of movement

RETURN

1. Return to starting position
2. Inhale while lowering weight to starting position

Misstep

Your low back is not against the pad.

Correction

Slide back on the seat until your low back is against the pad.

Misstep

You hold your breath during the sticking point.

Correction

Begin to exhale as soon as the bar nears the extended-elbow position.

The most common error made during the shoulder press is the tendency to arch the low back when the sticking point is reached. The back should be kept flat against the pad because the arched position inappropriately stresses the low back. Concentrate on keeping your buttocks and low back pressed against the pad.

*UPRIGHT ROW

If you are an experienced lifter who wants to add a second shoulder exercise to your program, consider adding the *upright row. Also, if you find that the first plate on the machine for the seated or shoulder press is too heavy, you can substitute the *upright row, using an empty bar.

The *upright row also develops the deltoids, but it differs from other shoulder exercises because it uses a pulling motion and does not involve the triceps muscle. This exercise can be performed using a barbell, dumbbells, or the low-pulley station on a machine. Figure 5.4 shows a lifter using a barbell.

Grip the barbell in an overhand grip, with hands 2 to 4 inches (5 to 10 centimeters) apart (figure 5.4*a*). Stand with your torso erect, arms straight, and feet shoulder-width apart. Rest the bar on your thighs. (See step 1, page 7, for more information on lifting the bar from the floor to the thighs.)

Pull the bar up along your abdomen and chest (figure 5.4*b*). Keep your elbows higher than your wrists and point them out to the sides. Pull the bar up until your elbows are at shoulder height. Exhale as the bar nears your shoulders. Pause briefly at the top of the movement.

Inhale as you begin to lower the bar to the starting position (figure 5.4*c*). Lower the bar in a smooth, steady, slow motion. Pause at the bottom of the movement before beginning the next rep.

Figure 5.4   ***Upright Row (Free Weight)**

PREPARATION

1. Use an overhand grip
2. Place hands 2 to 4 inches apart
3. Hold torso erect
4. Place feet shoulder-width apart
5. Keep arms straight
6. Rest bar on thighs

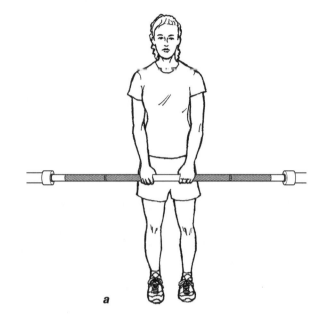

a

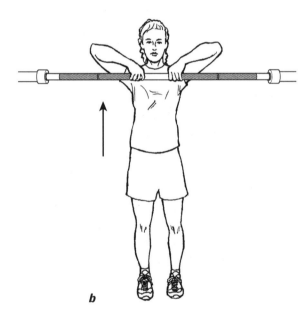

b

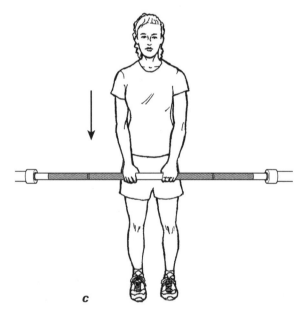

c

LIFT

1. Pull bar upward along abdomen and chest
2. Point elbows out
3. Keep elbows higher than wrists
4. Pull until elbows reach shoulder height
5. Exhale as bar nears shoulders
6. Pause briefly at top position

LOWER

1. Inhale as bar starts down
2. Lower bar slowly and smoothly
3. Pause at bottom of movement

Misstep

You allow your elbows to drop below your wrists.

Correction

Keep your elbows high and pointed up as you raise the bar.

Misstep

You allow the bar to drop too quickly back to the starting position.

Correction

Pause at the top position, then slowly return the bar to the starting position.

Shoulder Drill 1. *Choose One Exercise*

After reading about the characteristics and techniques of the exercises and the type of equipment required for each, you are ready to put this information to use. Consider the availability of equipment and access to spotters in your situation, then select one of the following exercises to use in your program:

- Standing press (free weight)
- Seated press (multi- or single-unit machine)
- Shoulder press (cam machine)

Write your shoulder exercise choice on the workout chart in the "Exercise" column (see page 126). If you intend to include the free-weight *upright row, record it on the workout chart immediately after the previously selected shoulder exercise.

Success Check

- Consider availability of equipment.
- Consider need for spotter and the availability of qualified people.
- Consider time available.
- Choose a shoulder exercise and record it on the workout chart.

Shoulder Drill 2. *Warm-Up and Trial Loads for Basic Exercises*

The next practice procedure answers the question "How much weight or load should I use?" Using the coefficient associated with the shoulder exercise you selected and the formula shown in figure 5.5, determine the trial load. (See step 2, pages 18-20, for more information on using this formula.) Round your results to the nearest 5-pound (2.25-kilogram) increment or to the closest weight-stack plate. Be sure to use the coefficient assigned to the exercise you selected. Use one-half of the amount determined for the trial load for your warm-up load in the exercise. These loads will be used in drills 4 and 5.

Success Check

- Determine your trial load by multiplying your body weight by the correct coefficient.
- Determine your warm-up load by dividing the trial load by two.
- Round off your trial and warm-up loads to the nearest 5-pound increment or to the closest weight-stack plate.
- Write down your warm-up and trial loads.

Calculations of Warm-Up and Trial Loads for Shoulder Exercises

Body weight	(Exercise)		Coefficient		Trial load	Warm-up load
		Female				
BWT = _____	(FW–standing press)	×	.22	=	_____	_____
BWT = _____	(C–shoulder press)	×	.25	=	_____	_____
BWT = _____	(M–seated press)	×	.15	=	_____	_____
		Male				
BWT = _____	(FW–standing press)	×	.38	=	_____	_____
BWT = _____	(C–shoulder press)	×	.40	=	_____	_____
BWT = _____	(M–seated press)	×	.35	=	_____	_____

BWT = body weight, FW = free weight, C = cam, M = multi- or single-unit machine exercise.

Note: If you are a male who weighs more than 175 lbs. (79 kg), record your body weight as 175 (79). If you are a female who weighs more than 140 lbs. (63.5 kg), record your body weight as 140 (63.5).

Figure 5.5 Warm-up and trial load determination for basic shoulder exercises.

Shoulder Drill 3. *Determine Trial Load for *Upright Row*

If you are an experienced lifter who has decided to add the *upright row, follow the directions to determine your trial load. (See step 2, pages 18-20, for more information.)

Based on your previous experience and knowledge of the weight that you can lift, select a weight that will allow you to perform 12 to 15 reps. Calculate the warm-up load by multiplying the trial load by .6, and round off the number to the nearest 5-pound increment or to the closest weight-stack plate (figure 5.6). These loads will be used in drill 4.

Success Check

- Select a weight that will allow 12 to 15 reps.
- Determine the warm-up load by multiplying the trial load by .6.
- Round off the warm-up load to the nearest 5-pound increment or to the closest weight-stack plate.
- Write down your warm-up and trial loads.

Calculation of Warm-Up Load for Additional Exercise

Exercise	Estimated trial load for 12-15 reps			Warm-up load
*Upright row	_____	× .6	=	_____

Figure 5.6 Formula for determining the warm-up load for the upright row.

Shoulder Drill 4. *Practice Proper Technique*

In this procedure, you are to perform 15 reps with the warm-up load determined in drill 2 (standing press, seated press, or shoulder press) or drill 3 (*upright row). If you are an experienced lifter who has decided to add the *upright row, practice it last.

Review the illustrations and instructions for the exercise, focusing on proper grip and body positioning. Visualize the movement pattern through the full range of motion. Inhale when you are ready to execute the exercise, then perform the movement with a slow, controlled velocity, remembering to exhale through the sticking point. Ask a qualified lifter to observe and assess your technique.

If you selected the free-weight standing press, you need a spotter. You also need to practice the skills of spotting this exercise. Identify a spotter with whom you will take turns completing the drill.

Instead of performing 15 reps in a continuous manner, rack the bar after each repetition for practice. Alternate responsibilities so that you and your partner both have a chance to develop the proper techniques for performing and spotting this exercise. Ask a qualified person to observe and assess your performance in the basic techniques.

Success Check

- For the standing press, all rackings are correctly performed.
- For all exercises, movement pattern, velocity, and breathing are correct.

Shoulder Drill 5. *Determine Training Load*

This practice procedure will help you determine an appropriate training load designed to produce 12 to 15 reps. For basic exercises, perform as many reps as possible with the calculated trial load from drill 2. Make sure that you execute the reps correctly.

If you executed 12 to 15 reps with the trial load, then your trial load is your training load. Record this number as your training load for this exercise on the workout chart (see page 126). If you did not perform 12 to 15 reps, go to drill 6 to make adjustments to the load.

Success Check

- Check for correct load.
- Maintain proper and safe technique during each rep.

Shoulder Drill 6. *Make Needed Load Adjustments*

If you performed fewer than 12 reps with your trial load, it is too heavy and you need to lighten it. On the other hand, if you performed more than 15 reps, the trial load is too light and you need to increase it. Use table 5.1 to determine the adjustment you need to make. Figure 5.7 shows the formula for making load adjustments.

Success Check

- Check correct use of load-adjustment chart (table 5.1).
- Record your training load on the workout chart (see page 126).

Table 5.1   Load Adjustments

Reps completed	Adjustments (lbs.)
< 7	−15
8-9	−10
10-11	−5
16-17	+5
18-19	+10
> 20	+15

Adjustments of Training Load		
Trial load	Adjustment	Training load
_____ +	_____ =	_____

Figure 5.7   Making adjustments to the training load for shoulder exercises.

SUCCESS SUMMARY FOR SHOULDER EXERCISES

This step involved selecting one shoulder exercise for which you have the needed equipment, and perhaps one more if you have already been training. Using a proper grip; the correct body position, movement, and breathing patterns; and accurate warm-up and training loads will ensure a positive outcome.

Once you have determined your training load and recorded it on your workout chart, you are ready to move on to step 6. In this step you will select exercises that are designed for developing the arms, including three for the front of the arm (the biceps curl, preacher curl, and *concentration curl) and three for the back of the arm (the two triceps-extension and triceps push-down exercises).

Before Taking the Next Step

Honestly answer each of the following questions. If you answer yes to all of the questions relevant to your level and exercise selection, you are ready to move on to step 6.

1. Have you selected a basic shoulder exercise? If you are an advanced lifter, do you want to add the *upright row?

2. Have you recorded your exercise selection (or selections) on the workout chart?

3. Have you determined a warm-up and training load for the exercise(s) you selected?

4. Have you recorded the warm-up and training loads on the workout chart?

5. Have you learned the proper technique for performing the exercise(s) you selected?

6. If the exercise(s) you selected require a spotter, have you identified a qualified person? Have you learned the proper spotting techniques?

Arm Exercises

Exercises that develop the upper arm are very popular, especially with beginning weight trainers. These muscles respond quickly when properly trained, and changes in this muscle area are noticed sooner and more often than changes in other body parts. The anterior and posterior portions of the upper arm are known as the biceps (the traditional "show me your muscle" muscle admired by many) and the triceps, respectively.

The free-weight biceps curl or *concentration curl, the preacher curl using the cam-type machine, and the low-pulley biceps curl using a single- or multi-unit weight machine are ideal exercises to develop the front of the upper arm.

They also develop the muscles in the front of the forearm.

The free-weight standing triceps extension or *supine triceps extension, the triceps extension using the cam machine, and the push-down on a multi- or single-unit weight machine are excellent exercises for developing the back of the upper arms.

When properly developed, the biceps and triceps muscles contribute to elbow-joint stabilization and, to a lesser extent, shoulder stabilization (long head of both biceps and triceps). Development of these muscles contributes to activities that require pulling (biceps) or pushing and throwing motions (triceps).

BICEPS EXERCISES

If you have access to free weights, you may select the biceps curl or the *concentration curl to develop the front of your upper arms. If you have access to either a cam or multi- or single-unit machine, you may select the preacher curl or the low-pulley biceps curl exercise.

Biceps Curl

To get in the preparation position, grasp the bar in an underhand grip with the hands about shoulder-width apart and evenly spaced (figure 6.1a). Hold your upper arms against your ribs and perpendicular to the floor with your elbows fully extended. The bar should touch the fronts of your thighs in this position. Your back should be straight, your eyes should be looking straight ahead, and your knees should be slightly flexed to reduce stress on the low back.

Misstep

Your elbows are slightly flexed in the preparatory position.

Correction

Stand erect with your shoulders back and your elbows extended.

Begin the execution phase by pulling the bar upward toward your shoulders, keeping your elbows and upper arms perpendicular to the floor and close to your sides (figure 6.1b). Avoid allowing your elbows and upper arms to move back or out to the sides. Your body must remain straight and erect throughout the exercise—no rocking, swinging, or jerking should occur. Begin to exhale as the bar nears your shoulders (sticking point).

Misstep

Your upper arms move back as you lift the bar.

Correction

Squeeze the insides of your upper arms against your ribs.

After flexing the elbows as far as possible, inhale as you slowly lower the bar to your thighs (figure 6.1c). Your elbows should be fully extended and you should pause momentarily at the thighs between each rep. Pause long enough to watch your elbows extend before curling the bar upward.

Figure 6.1   Biceps Curl (Free Weight)

PREPARATION

1. Use an underhand grip, hands shoulder-width apart
2. Hold torso erect
3. Hold head up, facing forward
4. Keep upper arms against ribs, elbows extended
5. Allow bar to touch fronts of thighs

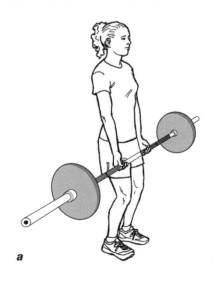

a

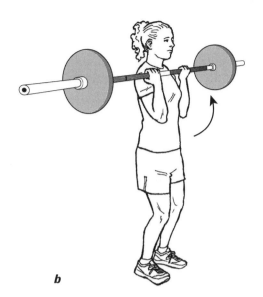

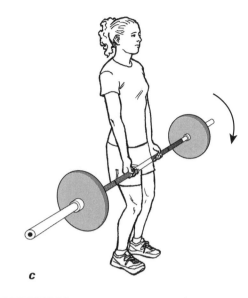

b

c

LIFT

1. Keep upper arms stationary
2. Keep elbows close to body
3. Curl bar to shoulders
4. Do not rock, jerk, or swing body
5. Begin to exhale as bar nears shoulders

RETURN

1. Inhale during downward movement
2. Lower bar slowly to thighs
3. Keep elbows close to sides
4. Extend arms completely

Misstep

You use momentum to complete the rep.

Correction

Keep your upper body erect. If this problem persists, stand with your back against the wall.

Misstep

Your wrists hyperextend (roll back) as you complete the rep.

Correction

Concentrate on keeping your wrists straight or slightly flexed.

Preacher Curl

For this biceps exercise option, assume a sitting position at a cam machine with your chest against the pad (figure 6.2a). Place your elbows on the pad in line with the axis of the cam, repositioning your arms if necessary. Adjust the seat so that your elbows are slightly lower than your shoulders.

Misstep

Your elbows are flexed at the start of the exercise.

Correction

Start the exercise with your elbows fully extended.

Grasp the handles in an underhand grip and begin the exercise at full elbow extension. Curl the handles upward as far as possible, pausing briefly at the top position (figure 6.2b). Exhale as the handles passes through the sticking point.

Inhale as you slowly lower the handles to the starting position, being careful not to allow the elbows to hyperextend (figure 6.2c). Remember, exhale when passing through the sticking point during the upward movement; inhale as you lower the handles.

Misstep

You use upper-torso movement to complete the curl.

Correction

Keep the chest against the pad and the elbows in line with the cams.

Figure 6.2 | Preacher Curl (Cam Machine)

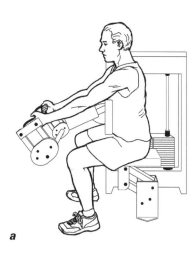
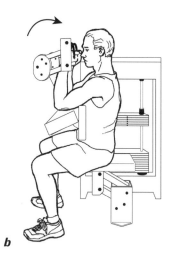
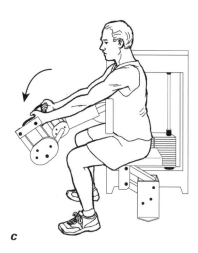

a   b   c

PREPARATION

1. Sit with chest against pad
2. Place elbows on pad in line with axis of cam
3. Adjust seat so that elbows are slightly lower than shoulders
4. Grasp handles with underhand grip

CURL

1. Curl upward as far as possible
2. Exhale through sticking point

RETURN

1. Inhale while slowly lowering handles to starting position
2. Do not allow elbows to hyperextend

Misstep

You do not go through the full range of motion.

Correction

Curl upward until your hands almost touch your shoulders. Lower until your elbows are fully extended.

Misstep

The weight drops too quickly.

Correction

Slowly lower the weight, being careful not to hyperextend your elbows.

Low-Pulley Biceps Curl

Assume a position facing the weight machine with your feet approximately 18 inches (46 centimeters) from it. Keep your torso erect, with your head up. Look at a point slightly above eye level. Keep your shoulders pulled back and your chest out. Your knees should be slightly flexed, your shoulders leaning back. If you begin with your knees locked, you will pull yourself forward as you pull the bar upward. Grasp the bar in an underhand grip and begin the exercise with the bar touching the front of the thighs and your elbows fully extended (figure 6.3a).

Misstep

Your elbows are flexed at the start.

Correction

Fully extend your elbows before starting and between each rep.

Curl the bar until it almost touches your shoulders (figure 6.3b). Avoid allowing your upper arms to move backward or out to the sides. Exhale as you pass through the sticking point and inhale while lowering the bar (figure 6.3c).

| **Figure 6.3** | **Low-Pulley Biceps Curl (Multi- or Single-Unit Machine)** |

PREPARATION

1. Hold torso erect
2. Slightly flex knees
3. Hold head up, eyes forward, shoulders back
4. Use underhand grip
5. Extend elbows fully
6. Rest bar on thighs

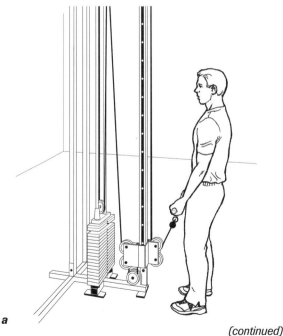

a

(continued)

Figure 6.3 *(continued)*

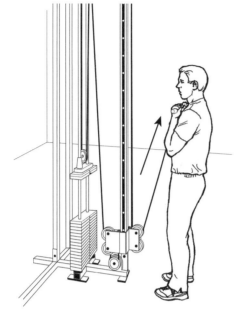

b

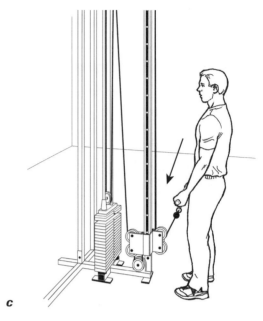

c

CURL

1. Pull bar to shoulder level
2. Keep upper arms stationary
3. Exhale as bar nears shoulders
4. Pause

LOWER

1. Slowly lower bar to starting position
2. Keep head up, eyes forward, shoulders back
3. Inhale when lowering bar

Misstep

You allow the weight plates to drop quickly to the weight stack.

Correction

Slowly lower the weight, allowing the plates to touch, not bang, against the stack.

Misstep

You do not go through the full range of motion.

Correction

Raise the bar until it almost touches your shoulders. Fully extend your elbows.

*Concentration Curl

A common supplementary exercise for the biceps is the *concentration curl. This exercise is similar to the free-weight biceps curl except that it is performed with one arm at a time using a dumbbell instead of a long bar.

The *concentration curl is often used to supplement other exercises for the front of the upper arm. The major muscle area involved is the same (biceps brachii).

Sit on a weight bench, feet wider than shoulder-width apart and flat on the floor. Lean your upper torso forward slightly. Grasp the dumbbell in one hand with an underhand grip. Straighten the arm to be worked and brace your upper arm against the side of your leg (figure 6.4a).

Slowly curl the dumbbell up toward your chin (figure 6.4b). Keep your upper torso stable, leaning slightly forward. Do not lean back as you curl the dumbbell toward your chin. Exhale as the dumbbell nears your chin. Pause at the top of the curl.

While maintaining the forward-lean position, slowly lower the weight to the starting position (figure 6.4c). Inhale as you lower the dumbbell.

Figure 6.4	*Concentration Curl (Free Weight)

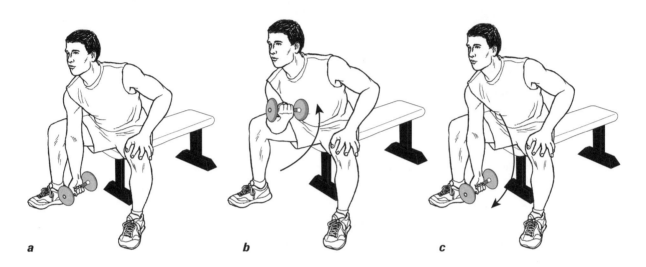

a   b   c

PREPARATION

1. Sit on bench
2. Lean upper torso forward
3. Place feet wider than shoulder-width apart and flat on floor
4. Grasp dumbbell in underhand grip
5. Hold arm straight, with upper arm braced against leg

CURL

1. Slowly curl dumbbell toward chin
2. Maintain stable forward-lean position
3. Exhale as dumbbell nears chin
4. Pause at full flexion

LOWER

1. Slowly lower dumbbell to starting position
2. Maintain forward-lean position
3. Inhale while lowering dumbbell

Misstep

You allow the dumbbell to drop quickly back to the starting position.

Correction

Slowly lower the dumbbell until the elbow is fully extended. Control the weight.

TRICEPS EXERCISES

If you have access to free weights, you may select the standing triceps extension or *supine triceps extension to develop the back of your upper arms. If you have access to either a cam or multi- or single-unit machine, select either the triceps extension or the triceps push-down.

Standing Triceps Extension

Hold the bar in a narrow overhand grip with hands about 6 inches (15 centimeters) apart. Use the fundamental lifting techniques presented in step 2 (see page 5) to take the bar from the floor to the shoulders, and those in step 5 (see page 56) to press the bar to a fully extended position overhead (figure 6.5a).

Misstep

Your hands are too far apart.

Correction

Space your hands no more than 6 inches (15 centimeters) apart on the bar.

Begin the execution phase by lowering the bar in a slow, controlled manner behind your head to shoulder level by flexing the elbows (figure 6.5b). Inhale while you lower the bar. The upper arms maintain a vertical position, elbows pointing straight up, as you lower the bar. As you lower it, think "lower" not "drop." Control the bar's downward momentum and pause with it at shoulder level before pushing upward.

From a fully flexed position, push the bar back to a fully extended position (figure 6.5c). During the upward movement, your elbows will have a tendency to move forward and bow out. Keep your upper arms close to your ears and your elbows pointing straight up. Exhale through the sticking point, which occurs as the bar approaches the top position. Do not move your legs or torso in any way to assist in moving the bar upward.

| Figure 6.5 | Standing Triceps Extension (Free Weight) |

Preparation

SPOTTER

1. Stand directly behind partner
2. Stand as close as possible without touching partner
3. Knuckles face forward
4. Place feet shoulder-width apart

LIFTER

1. Use overhand grip, hands 6 inches apart
2. Keep torso erect
3. Hold head up, facing forward
4. Place feet shoulder-width apart
5. Hold elbows close to ears, pointing straight up

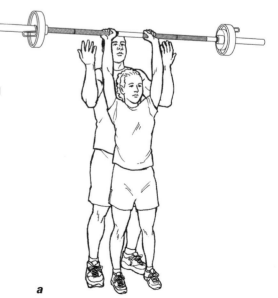

a

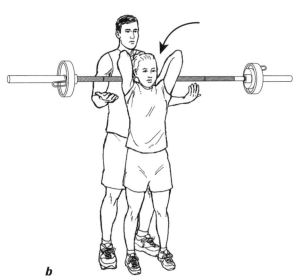
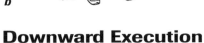

b

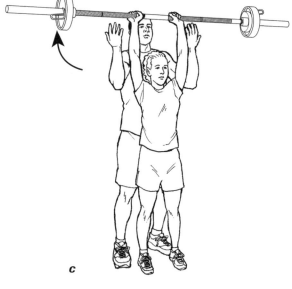

c

Downward Execution

SPOTTER

1. Keep hands close to bar, tracking downward movement
2. Watch for excessive bar speed

LIFTER

1. Lower bar behind head to top of shoulders
2. Keep elbows pointed up
3. Control downward movement
4. Inhale as bar is lowered

Upward Execution

SPOTTER

1. Keep hands close to bar, tracking upward movement
2. Assist only if necessary
3. Caution partner not to lean back or hold breath

LIFTER

1. Push bar to full extension
2. Keep elbows back, close to ears, pointing upward
3. Exhale as bar passes through sticking point

Misstep

Your elbows bow out away from your head.

Correction

Concentrate on keeping your upper arms close to your ears.

Misstep

You lower the bar only to the top of your head.

Correction

Perform the exercise in front of a mirror. Make sure you lower the bar to shoulder level during each rep.

As the spotter, you should stand directly behind your partner as close as you can without causing contact (figure 6.5a). With your arms outstretched and your open hands under (but not touching) the bar, follow it as it moves up and down (figures 6.5b and c).

Most errors associated with the standing triceps extension involve moving the upper arms out of position. When using free weights, your elbows will tend to move forward and bow out during the upward phase. Concentrate on keeping your elbows close to your ears and pointing them straight up.

Triceps Extension

Assume a sitting position in the cam machine with your back firmly against the pad. Adjust the seat until your shoulders are close to the same height as your elbows. Your elbows should be in line with the axis of the cam. Adjust the position of your upper arms to align them if necessary. Place your hands, upper arms, and elbows on the pad (figure 6.6a).

From this position, push with your hands until your elbows are completely straight (figure 6.6b). Do not allow your upper arms to lift off the pads. Pause in the extended position, then slowly return to the starting position (figure 6.6c). Exhale while pushing through the sticking point and inhale during the return.

| Figure 6.6 | Triceps Extension (Cam Machine) |

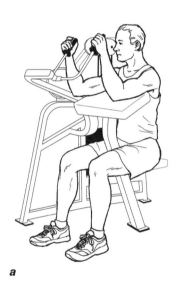
a

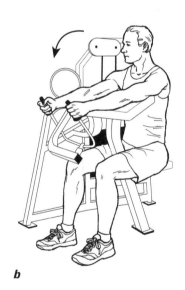
b

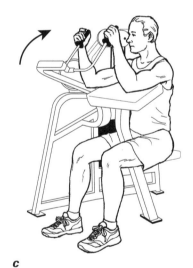
c

PREPARATION

1. Place back firmly against pad
2. Adjust seat so that shoulders are close to same height as elbows
3. Place upper arms and hands on pads

EXTEND

1. Extend elbows completely
2. Keep upper arms back, elbows pointing forward
3. Exhale through sticking point

RETURN

1. Slowly return to starting position
2. Inhale during return to starting position

Misstep

Your upper arms and elbows lift off the pads.

Correction

Keep pressing your upper arms and elbows against the pads. Lighten the load, if necessary.

Misstep

You do not breathe properly during the rep.

Correction

Exhale as you press down through the sticking point. Inhale during the return to the starting position.

Triceps Push-Down

Assume an erect position facing the weight machine, with your feet approximately shoulder-width apart. Grasp the lat bar in an overhand grip, with your hands no more than 6 inches (15 centimeters) apart (figure 6.7a). Begin the exercise with the bar at chest height and your upper arms pressed firmly against your ribs.

From this position extend your forearms until your elbows are straight and the bar touches your thighs (figure 6.7b). Be sure to extend your elbows completely. Pause, then slowly return the bar to chest height without moving your upper arms and torso (figure 6.7c). Exhale after passing the sticking point, and inhale during the return.

Misstep

Your upper arms move away from your ribs.

Correction

Squeeze your upper arms against your ribs. Pause at the fully extended and flexed elbow positions.

Figure 6.7   Triceps Push-Down (Multi- or Single-Unit Machine)

PREPARATION

1. Stand erect
2. Place feet shoulder-width apart
3. Use overhand grip
4. Place hands no more than 6 inches (15 centimeters) apart
5. Begin with bar at chest height
6. Squeeze upper arms against ribs

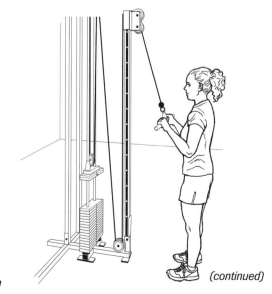

a

(continued)

Figure 6.7   (continued)

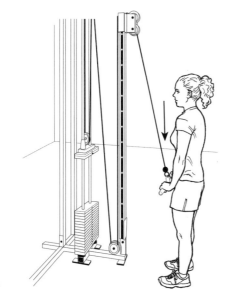

b

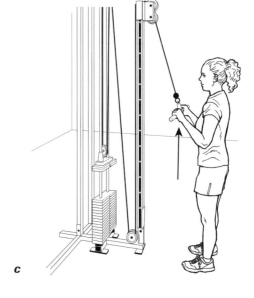

c

EXTEND

1. Extend elbows until bar touches thighs
2. Do not move upper arms or torso
3. Exhale when passing through sticking point
4. Pause

RETURN

1. Inhale while slowly returning bar to chest height
2. Keep wrists straight throughout exercise

Misstep

You allow the bar to move above the shoulders.

Correction

The bar should begin at chest height and not be allowed to move higher than shoulder level. Think, "Knuckles below the shoulders."

Misstep

Your torso moves back and forth.

Correction

Maintain a stable, upright position in which your head, shoulders, hips, and feet form a straight line. Lighten the load if necessary.

As you return the bar to chest height, take care not to move it too quickly. This causes many bar-location and arm-position errors and too much stress on the elbows, muscles, and joints. Slowly return the bar to chest height in a controlled fashion.

*Supine Triceps Extension

If you are an experienced lifter who is ready for a second triceps exercise, consider adding the *supine triceps extension. Like the standing triceps extension, this exercise requires a spotter. It is a pushing exercise that is performed lying down on your back, usually on a flat bench.

Lie on the bench and place your feet flat on the floor. Legs are flexed 90 degrees. Grip the bar in an overhand grip, hands evenly spaced about 8 inches (20 centimeters) apart (figure 6.8a). Maintain a stable, flat position on the bench.

Keeping the upper arms stationary, slowly lower the bar toward your head (figure 6.8b). Inhale as you lower the bar. Keep your elbows pointing straight up; do not allow them to bow out.

Extend the elbows and push the bar back to the starting position (figure 6.8c). Keep your elbows still; do not let them bow out. Exhale as the bar nears the top position.

Figure 6.8	*Supine Triceps Extension (Free Weight)

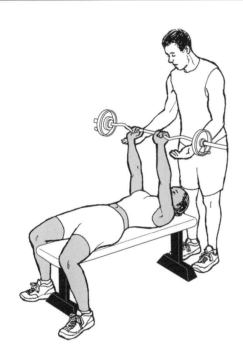

a

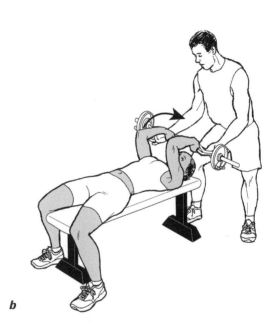

b

Preparation

SPOTTER

1. Stand at partner's head
2. Hand bar to partner

LIFTER

1. Use an overhand grip, hands evenly spaced 8 inches (20 centimeters) apart
2. Take a stable position, flat on bench
3. Flex legs 90 degrees
4. Place feet flat on floor

Downward Execution

SPOTTER

1. Keep hands under bar to protect partner's head
2. Help control downward speed of bar

LIFTER

1. Keep upper arms stationary
2. Keep elbows straight up
3. Do not allow elbows to bow out
4. Slowly lower bar
5. Inhale while lowering bar

(continued)

Figure 6.8 (continued)

Upward Execution

SPOTTER

1. Assist partner through sticking point if needed
2. Take weight after last repetition and return bar to floor

LIFTER

1. Push upward to extend elbows
2. Keep elbows pointed straight up
3. Keep elbows from bowing out
4. Exhale when near top position

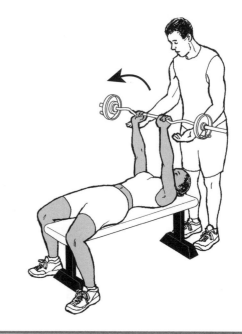

c

 Misstep

Your upper arms move out and forward.

Correction

Concentrate on keeping your upper arms stationary during the exercise.

 Misstep

Your elbows are not perpendicular to the floor at the beginning of each rep.

Correction

Concentrate on keeping your elbows pointing up.

As the spotter, you should stand forward of your partner's head about 2 to 6 inches (5 to 15 centimeters) from the bench (figure 6.8*a*). Using the technique described in step 1 (see page 4), grip the bar using a wide alternated grip, lift the bar off the floor, stand at your partner's head, and give her time to grasp the bar between your hands. At your partner's OK command, guide the bar to a straight-elbow position over her chest. Before releasing the bar, be sure that your partner's elbows are completely straight. Practice making the handoff as smooth as possible. If your handoff is too far forward or back, it will disturb your partner's stable position on the bench, which may contribute to a poor performance or injury.

Follow the downward motion of the bar with your open hands and eyes (figure 6.8*b*). Follow the bar back up to the starting position (figure 6.8*c*). As your partner's elbows straighten during the last repetition and after she has given the OK signal, assist by grasping the bar and returning it to the floor.

Arm Drill 1.   *Choose Two Exercises*

After reading about the characteristics and techniques involved in the exercises and the type of equipment required for each, you are ready to put what you have learned to use. Consider the availability of equipment and your situation, then select one biceps exercise and one triceps exercise to use in your program:

Biceps

- Biceps curl (free weight)
- Preacher curl (cam machine)
- Low-pulley biceps curl (multi- or single-unit machine)

Triceps

- Standing triceps extension (free weight)
- Triceps extension (cam machine)
- Triceps push-down (multi- or single-unit machine)

Write your two arm exercise choices on the workout chart in the "Exercise" column (see page 126). If you intend to include the free-weight *concentration curl (biceps) or free-weight *supine triceps extension (triceps), record it on the workout chart immediately after the arm exercises already selected.

Success Check

- Consider availability of equipment.
- Consider need for a spotter and the availability of qualified people.
- Consider time available.
- Choose two arm exercises and record them on the workout chart.

Arm Drill 2.   *Warm-Up and Trial Loads for Basic Exercises*

This practice procedure will answer the question "How much weight or load should I use?" Using the coefficients associated with the arm exercises you selected and the formulas shown in figure 6.9, determine the trial load. (See step 2, pages 18-20, for more information on using this formula.) Round your results to the nearest 5-pound (2.25-kilogram) increment or to the closest weight-stack plate. Be sure to use the coefficient assigned to the exercise you selected. Use one-half of the amount determined for the trial load for your warm-up load in the exercise. These loads will be used in drills 4 and 5.

Success Check

- Determine your trial load by multiplying your body weight by the correct coefficient.
- Determine your warm-up load by dividing the trial load by two.
- Round off your trial and warm-up loads to the nearest 5-pound increment or to the closest weight-stack plate.
- Write down your warm-up and trial loads.

Calculations of Warm-Up and Trial Loads for Arm Exercises

Biceps

Body weight	(Exercise)		Coefficient		Trial load	Warm-up load
		Female				
BWT = _____	(FW–biceps curl)	×	.23	=	_____	_____
BWT = _____	(C–preacher curl)	×	.12	=	_____	_____
BWT = _____	(M–low-pulley biceps curl)	×	.15	=	_____	_____
		Male				
BWT = _____	(FW–biceps curl)	×	.30	=	_____	_____
BWT = _____	(C–preacher curl)	×	.20	=	_____	_____
BWT = _____	(M–low-pulley biceps curl)	×	.25	=	_____	_____

Triceps

Body weight	(Exercise)		Coefficient		Trial load	Warm-up load
		Female				
BWT = _____	(FW–standing triceps extension)	×	.12	=	_____	_____
BWT = _____	(C–triceps extension)	×	.13	=	_____	_____
BWT = _____	(M–triceps push-down)	×	.19	=	_____	_____
		Male				
BWT = _____	(FW–standing triceps extension)	×	.21	=	_____	_____
BWT = _____	(C–triceps extension)	×	.35	=	_____	_____
BWT = _____	(M–triceps push-down)	×	.32	=	_____	_____

BWT = body weight, FW = free weight, C = cam, M = multi- or single-unit machine exercise.

Note: If you are a male who weighs more than 175 lbs. (79 kg), record your body weight as 175 (79). If you are a female who weighs more than 140 lbs. (63.5 kg), record your body weight as 140 (63.5).

Figure 6.9 Warm-up and trial load determination for basic arm exercises.

Arm Drill 3. *Determine Trial Loads for *Concentration Curl and *Supine Triceps Extension*

If you are an experienced lifter who wants to add the *concentration curl or the *supine triceps extension, follow the directions to determine your trial load. (See step 2, pages 18-20, for more information.)

Based on your previous experience and knowledge of the weight that you can lift, select a weight that will allow you to perform 12 to 15 reps. Calculate the warm-up load by multiplying the trial load by .6, and round off the number to the nearest 5-pound increment (figure 6.10). These loads will be used in drill 4.

Calculation of Warm-Up Load
for Additional Exercise

Exercise	Estimated trial load for 12-15 reps				Warm-up load
*Concentration curl	_____	×	.6	=	_____
*Supine triceps extension	_____	×	.6	=	_____

Figure 6.10   Formula for determining the warm-up load for the *concentration curl and the *supine triceps extension.

Success Check

- Select a weight that will allow 12 to 15 reps.
- Determine the warm-up load by multiplying the trial load by .6.

- Round off the warm-up load to the nearest 5-pound increment.
- Write down your warm-up and trial loads.

Arm Drill 4.   *Practice Proper Technique*

In this procedure you are to perform 15 reps with the warm-up load determined in drill 2 (biceps curl, preacher curl, or low-pulley biceps curl for the biceps; standing triceps extension, triceps extension, or triceps push-down for the triceps) or drill 3 (*concentration curl for the biceps, *supine triceps extension for the triceps). If you are an experienced lifter who has decided to add the *concentration curl or the *supine triceps extension, practice it last.

Review the illustrations and instructions for the exercise, focusing on proper grip and body positioning. Visualize the movement pattern through the full range of motion. Inhale when you are ready to execute the exercise, then perform the movement with a slow, controlled velocity, remembering to exhale through the sticking point. Check your technique either by watching yourself in a mirror or by asking a qualified lifter to observe and assess your technique.

If you selected the free-weight standing triceps extension or the *supine triceps extension, you need a spotter. You also need to practice the skills of spotting these exercises. Identify a spotter with whom you will take turns completing the drill.

Instead of performing 15 reps in a continuous manner, return the bar to the floor after each repetition to practice getting in the right spotting position and properly handling the bar. Alternate responsibilities so that you and your partner both have a chance to develop the techniques that are required in performing and spotting these exercises. Ask a qualified person to observe and assess your performance in the basic techniques.

Success Check

- For the *supine triceps extension, all bar handoffs and bar returns are correctly performed.
- For all exercises, movement pattern, velocity, and breathing are correct.

Arm Drill 5.   *Determine Training Load*

This practice procedure will help you determine an appropriate training load designed to produce 12 to 15 reps. For basic exercises, perform as many reps as possible with the calculated trial load from drill 2. Make sure that the reps are correctly executed.

If you executed 12 to 15 reps with your trial load, then your trial load is your training load. Record this number as your training load for this exercise in the workout chart (see page 126). If you did not perform 12 to 15 reps, go to drill 6 to make adjustments to the load.

Success Check

• Check for correct load.

• Maintain proper and safe technique during each rep.

Arm Drill 6.   *Make Needed Load Adjustments*

If you performed fewer than 12 reps with your trial load, the load is too heavy and you need to lighten it. On the other hand, if you performed more than 15 reps, it is too light and you need to increase it. Use table 6.1 to determine the adjustment you need to make. Figure 6.11 shows the formula for making load adjustments.

Success Check

• Check correct use of load adjustment chart (table 6.1).

• Record your training load on the workout chart (see page 126).

Table 6.1   Load Adjustments

Reps completed	Adjustments (lbs.)
<7	−15
8-9	−10
10-11	−5
16-17	+5
18-19	+10
>20	+15

Adjustments of Training Load

Trial load	Adjustment	Training load
_____ +	_____ =	_____

Figure 6.11   Making adjustments to the training load for arm exercises.

SUCCESS SUMMARY FOR ARM EXERCISES

This step involved selecting one arm exercise for the biceps and another for the triceps for which you have the needed equipment, and perhaps one more for each if you have already been training. Using a proper grip; the correct body position, movement, and breathing patterns; and accurate warm-up and training loads will ensure a positive outcome.

Before Taking the Next Step

Honestly answer each of the following questions. If you answer yes to all of the questions relevant to your level and exercise selection, you are ready to move on to step 7.

1. Have you selected basic biceps and triceps exercises? If you are an advanced lifter, do you want to add the *concentration curl (biceps) or *supine triceps extension (triceps)?

2. Have you recorded your exercise selections on the workout chart?

3. Have you determined warm-up and training loads for the exercises you selected?

4. Have you recorded the warm-up and training loads on the workout chart?

5. Have you learned the proper technique for performing the exercises you selected?

6. If an exercise you selected requires a spotter, have you identified a qualified person? Have you learned the proper spotting techniques?

Once you have determined your training load and recorded it on your workout chart, you are ready to move on to step 7. In step 7 you will select exercises (classified as either multijoint or single-joint) that are designed for developing the legs. The multijoint exercises in this step are the free-weight lunge, machine leg press, and *back squat; the single-joint exercise options are the *knee extension, *knee curl, and *standing heel raise.

Leg Exercises

Exercises that develop the upper legs are considered very demanding physically due to the large muscle area involved. The area of the body worked by these exercises is sometimes referred to as the *power zone*. These muscle groups, the largest in the body—quadriceps (front of the thigh), hamstrings (back of the thigh), and gluteal muscles (the buttocks)—are responsible for our ability to run, jump, and make quick starts and fast stops, as well as quick lateral, backward, pushing, pulling, rotating, and kicking movements. They also stabilize the upper body during most of its movements. The importance of developing these muscle groups is obvious, and they must not be neglected in favor of the more visible muscles of the upper body.

The exercises in this step can be classified as either multi- or single-joint. The multijoint exercises are the free-weight lunge, machine leg press, and *back squat (free weight). These exercises are excellent for developing the quadriceps, hamstrings, and the hips and buttocks.

Some additional exercises involve only one joint (single-joint exercises), focusing on one primary muscle group or body-part area. The machine *knee extension trains the quadriceps; the machine *knee curl, the hamstrings; and the free weight *standing heel raise, the back of the lower legs (the calves).

If you have access to free weights, you may select the lunge or the *back squat to develop your legs. To isolate your calves, add the *standing heel raise. If you have access to either a cam machine or a multi- or single-unit machine, try the leg press.

MULTIJOINT EXERCISES

Multijoint exercises require you to simultaneously extend the knee and hip joints. The quadriceps extend the knee joint, while the hamstrings flex the knee and, with the help of the gluteal muscles, also extend the hip joint.

The multijoint exercises featured in this step contribute to knee and hip-joint stabilization, muscle padding for protection of the hip, and lower-body sculpting. The leg and hip strength gained through these exercises is especially beneficial to those involved in athletic activities.

Lunge

Begin with your feet shoulder-width apart, eyes straight ahead, head up, shoulders back, chest out, and back straight (figure 7.1a). Do not lean your upper torso forward. This erect posture should be maintained throughout the exercise.

The forward execution phase begins with a slow, controlled step forward on your preferred leg (figure 7.1b). Be careful not to overstride. Lower your hips enough so that the top of your forward thigh is parallel to the floor and your forward knee is directly over your ankle (figure 7.1c). Your front foot should be straight ahead and your back knee somewhat flexed to stretch your hip-flexor muscles. The back knee should not quite touch the floor.

Push off your front foot and smoothly return to the starting position without using upper-torso momentum. Step forward with the other foot in the next rep and continue alternating until the set is completed. At first you might have to slide (stutter step) your foot on the floor in order to return to the starting position. As you gain strength and develop better balance, sliding your foot will not be necessary.

CAUTION The lunge is a relatively difficult exercise to perform because of the balance required. First try lunges without weights to develop the needed balance. When you feel comfortable with the forward and backward movements and with your balance, begin using dumbbells.

Figure 7.1 Lunge (Free Weight)

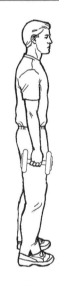
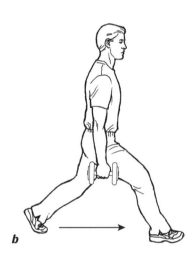
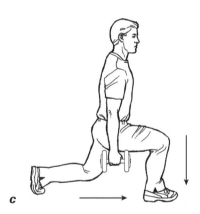

a   b   c

PREPARATION

1. Use an overhand grip with arms hanging straight down at sides
2. Hold torso erect, with head up and eyes straight forward
3. Place feet shoulder-width apart

STEP FORWARD

1. Keep upper torso erect
2. Inhale and take a slow, controlled step forward
3. Place front foot straight ahead

LOWER AND RETURN

1. Lower hips until front thigh is parallel to floor
2. Keep front knee over ankle
3. Moderately flex back knee, but do not let it touch floor
4. Exhale and push off with front foot to return to starting position
5. Maintain an erect torso
6. Keep eyes looking straight ahead

Misstep

Your front foot points laterally.

Correction

Practice stepping on a line. Form a straight line with the thigh, knee, and foot.

When first learning the lunge, you may tend to overstride. To avoid this, begin with small steps forward and gradually increase each stride until the thigh of the leading leg is parallel and the lower leg is perpendicular to the floor.

Leg Press

This exercise typically involves the use of a multi- or single-unit machine, although some equipment companies make a cam-type leg press machine. Begin by adjusting the seat so that your knees are flexed 90 degrees or less. If you have trouble, use a mirror or ask someone to help you establish a 90-degree angle. Your knees should be apart so that they are not pressed back into the abdomen and chest, which could create difficulty when you attempt to inhale. Sit erect, with your low back against the back of the seat, toes pointed slightly outward, and feet flat against the pedal surface

(figure 7.2a). Grasp the handrails to stabilize your body.

Initiate the forward execution phase by pushing your legs to the extended-knee position while maintaining an upright torso position (figure 7.2b). Your knees should press toward each other as they are extended. Avoid twisting your body as you extend your legs. Do not lock out your knees at any time. Exhale while pressing outward.

For the backward execution phase, allow your legs to move back toward your body as far as possible without lifting your buttocks off the seat or allowing the weight plate to touch the stack (figure 7.2c). Inhale as you return to the starting position. This movement should be performed in a very slow, controlled manner. Allowing the weights to drop quickly back toward the weight stack and stopping them just before they hit could cause injury to your low back.

| **Figure 7.2** | **Leg Press (Multi- or Single–Unit Machine)** |

PREPARATION

1. Hold torso erect, back against back of seat
2. Flex legs 90 degrees or less
3. Place feet flat on pedal surface in a parallel position
4. Grasp handrails with arms straight

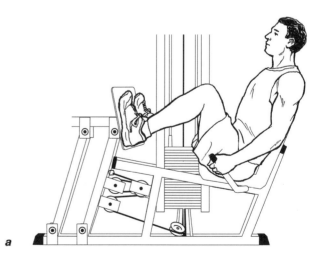

a

(continued)

Figure 7.2 (continued)

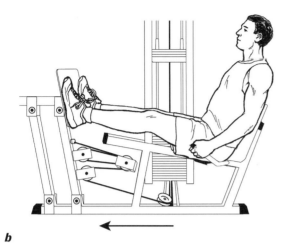

b

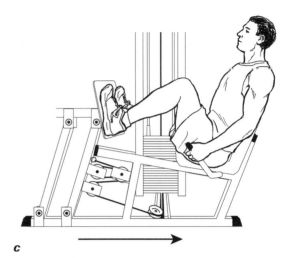

c

PUSH

1. Push the pedals away, extending knees
2. Maintain erect body position
3. Do not lock knees out
4. Avoid twisting body
5. Exhale during push

BACKWARD EXECUTION

1. Slowly return legs to 90-degree flexion
2. Maintain erect body position
3. Inhale as knees flex

Misstep

Your feet are not flat on the pedal surface.

Correction

Think about pushing with the middle or back half of your foot.

Misstep

Your torso leans forward.

Correction

Sit with your back and hips pushed against the seat.

Most errors associated with the leg press involve the speed of extension and flexion and locking the knees. Many lifters have a tendency to press out too quickly, causing the knees to lock out. The danger is that you might hyperextend your knees and cause injury. Control your forward speed and concentrate on stopping just before your knees lock out.

Another common error is letting the foot pedal weight free-fall back to the starting position. The first step in correcting errors is to slowly extend the knees, then make a slow, controlled movement back to the starting position.

*Back Squat

The final multijoint exercise is the *back squat. This exercise targets all the major muscle groups of the lower body—quadriceps, hamstrings, and gluteal muscles. In addition, many upper-body muscles are recruited to achieve an upright, flat-back (not rounded or hunched over) position, keep the bar in place on the shoulder, and provide protective support for the low back.

The *back squat is a more advanced exercise because of the upright, flat-back position (required to minimize stress on the low back), the placement of the barbell across the shoulders and upper back, and the balance needed throughout the whole exercise. A spotter is required. A common strategy when first learning how to perform this exercise is to try it with a long broomstick to develop the needed body position, bar placement, and overall balance. Once you have mastered the correct technique, progress to an empty bar, then to a bar with weight plates. Be sure to use collars.

Stand in the rack with feet flat on the floor, slightly wider than shoulder-width apart (figure 7.3a). Grasp the bar in an overhand grip, with hands slightly wider than shoulder-width apart. With the help of the spotter, position the bar across your shoulders at the base of your neck. Keep your hips directly under the bar, chest out, shoulders back, and head up.

Misstep

The bar is positioned too high on your neck.

Correction

Place the bar on your shoulders at the base of your neck. You should be able to keep your head up even with the bar across your shoulders.

For the downward execution phase, slowly squat (figure 7.3b). Do not lean too far forward. Keep your feet flat on the floor and your knees aligned with your feet. Inhale as you descend. Continue to descend until your thighs are parallel to the floor.

Begin the upward movement with your legs first (figure 7.3c). Keep your head up and chest out. Exhale at the sticking point as you straighten your hips and knees and return to the starting position.

Figure 7.3   *Back Squat (Free Weight)

Preparation

SPOTTER

1. Stand directly behind and close to partner
2. Place hands close to bar
3. Keep back flat and knees slightly flexed
4. Assist only if necessary

LIFTER

1. Use an overhand grip, hands slightly wider than shoulder-width
2. Position bar on shoulders at base of neck
3. Align hips directly under bar, with chest out, shoulders back, head up
4. Position feet flat on floor slightly wider than shoulder-width

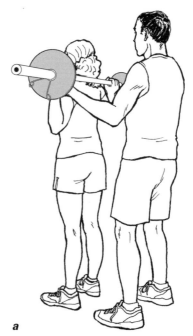

a

(continued)

Figure 7.3 *(continued)*

Squat

SPOTTER

1. Squat with partner
2. Track bar with both hands

LIFTER

1. Squat slowly
2. Avoid excessive forward lean
3. Keep feet flat on floor, knees in line with feet
4. Continue squatting until your thighs are parallel to floor
5. Inhale on descent

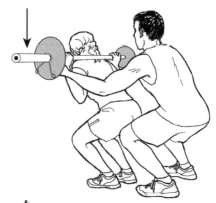

b

Rise

SPOTTER

1. Ascend with partner
2. Keep hands close to bar
3. Assist only when necessary

LIFTER

1. Begin movement with legs first
2. Keep head up and chest out
3. Straighten hips and knees
4. Exhale during sticking point

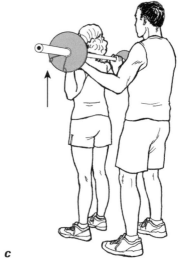

c

Rack the Bar

SPOTTER

1. Walk with partner until bar is racked
2. Tell partner when bar is safely racked

LIFTER

1. Walk forward until bar contacts rack
2. Squat down until bar is in rack
3. Never lean forward to rack bar

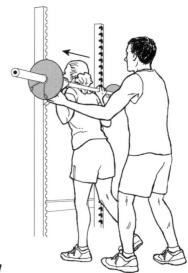

d

Misstep

You lower your head to look at the floor.

Correction

Focus your eyes straight ahead or slightly up. Do not look up at the ceiling, however. This will help you maintain balance.

Misstep

You allow your knees to move in front of your feet.

Correction

Keep your heels on the floor and use a shallower squatting depth.

As the spotter, you should stand directly behind your partner as close as you can without causing contact (figure 7.3a). To assist your partner in removing the bar from the rack, grasp it with a pronated grip between her hands and shoulders (or wider than her hands). At the lifter's OK command, carefully help her to lift the bar off the supports and take a step backward as she also steps backward to clear the supports. Take a hip-width stance and a flat-back body position. Before releasing the bar, be sure that your partner has the bar under control. Practice this procedure so that you can provide assistance without bumping your partner or placing your feet where hers will be—either error could cause her to lose her balance or drop the bar.

Once the downward phase begins, squat with the lifter and follow the bar's path with your open hands (figure 7.3b). Be sure to maintain the flat-back body position. During the upward phase, ascend with your open hands still under the bar (figure 7.3c).

As you ascend with the lifter following the last repetition, prepare to help rack the bar. After your partner gives the OK signal, assist by grasping the bar and walking forward with her to rack it (figure 7.3d). Be sure that the bar is resting on the shelf of the supports before releasing it.

Misstep

You lean forward to rack the bar.

Correction

Walk straight ahead to the rack and squat down to rack the bar. Maintain a flat-back position.

SINGLE-JOINT EXERCISES

If you are an experienced lifter who is ready for a more challenging leg program, consider one or more additional leg exercises. At first choose one of the single-joint exercises to complement the multijoint exercise you are already performing. A common approach is to add the machine *knee extension and machine *knee curl exercises to a program that already includes either the free-weight lunge or the machine leg press. Later, as you become even more trained, consider replacing the lunge or leg press with the free-weight *back squat exer-

cise. The *standing heel raise exercise can be added at any time.

*Knee Extension

This exercise places a localized stress on the quadriceps muscle group. You perform it by extending your knees while sitting in a cam machine with ankle or lower-leg pad(s) positioned across the instep of your feet.

Sit in the cam machine (figure 7.4a). Keep your torso erect and your low back flat against

95

the back of the seat. Look straight ahead and keep your head up. Tuck your shins and ankles behind the pads. Grasp the edge of the table, chair, or the handles of the machine.

Slowly extend your legs (figure 7.4b). Be sure to go through the complete range of motion. Exhale as you extend your legs. Pause briefly at the top position.

Slowly lower the weight and return to the starting position (figure 7.4c). Do not rise out of the seat. Keep a firm grip on the table, chair, or handles to keep the buttocks in contact with the seat. Inhale as you lower the weight. Control the weight as you lower it, and do not allow it to crash into the weight stack. Pause at the bottom position before beginning the next repetition.

Figure 7.4   *Knee Extension (Cam Machine)

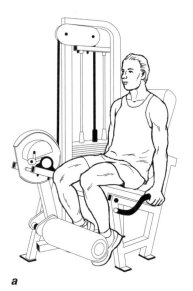

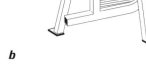

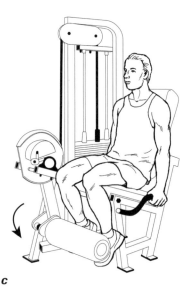

a

b

c

PREPARATION

1. Assume a sitting position
2. Grip edge of table, chair, or handles
3. Keep torso erect, low back flat
4. Hold head up, facing forward
5. Place shins and ankles behind pads

EXTEND

1. Slowly extend lower leg through complete range of motion
2. Exhale while extending
3. Pause briefly in extended position

LOWER

1. Slowly lower weight
2. Keep buttocks in contact with seat
3. Pause at bottom position
4. Do not allow weight plate to hit weight stack
5. Inhale while lowering weight

*Knee Curl

This exercise specifically stresses the hamstrings muscle group. You perform it by flexing the knees while lying face down on a cam machine with ankle or lower-leg pads positioned across your heels and Achilles tendons.

Lie down on the cam machine and grip the handles or the bench (figure 7.5a). Keep your hips and chest in contact with the bench at all times. Your knees should be just below the edge of the bench. Tuck your ankles under the pads so that they rest against your Achilles tendons.

Curl your legs, flexing your knees and bringing your heels as close to your buttocks as you can (figure 7.5b). Exhale as you curl your legs.

Pause briefly at the top of the upward movement.

Control the weight as you slowly lower it to the starting position (figure 7.5c). Keep your hips and chest in contact with the bench by firmly gripping the handles or sides of the bench. Inhale as you lower the weight.

Figure 7.5 *Knee Curl (Cam Machine)

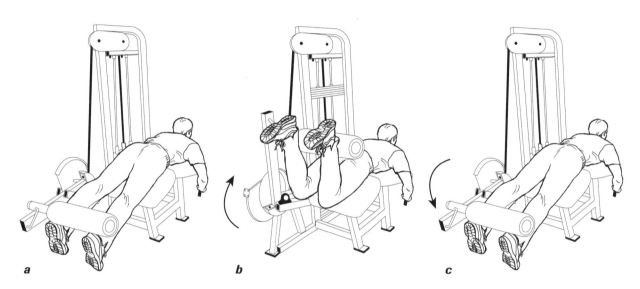

a

b

c

PREPARATION

1. Assume a prone position
2. Grip handles or edge of bench
3. Keep hips flat, chest on bench
4. Position knees below edge of bench
5. Place ankles under pads

CURL

1. Flex knees as much as possible by lifting heels toward buttocks
2. Do not allow hips to rise off bench
3. Exhale during upward movement
4. Pause briefly in fully flexed position

RETURN

1. Lower weight slowly
2. Keep chest on bench
3. Inhale during downward movement

Misstep

You allow the weight to drop quickly as you return to the starting position.

Correction

Control the speed of the downward phase and minimize the force of the plates as they hit the weight stack. Do not crash the plates onto the stack.

*Standing Heel Raise

This pushing exercise uses plantar flexion at the ankle joint to train the calf muscles, the soleus and gastrocnemius. The standing heel raise can be performed with a barbell across the shoulders, with one or two dumbbells (as shown in figure 7.6), or with your body weight only.

Begin by finding a stable surface to stand on. You need an elevated surface, about 6 inches (15 centimeters) high, that will not move as you perform the exercise. A shallow step is ideal. To help you learn the balance needed to perform the exercise correctly, do a few repetitions using only your body weight before adding the barbell or dumbbells.

Place the bar on your shoulders or hold a dumbbell in each hand (figure 7.6a). Place your feet hip-width apart, with the balls of both feet near the edge of the elevated surface. Keep your torso erect while leaning slightly forward and keeping your knees straight. Your eyes should focus straight ahead to help you maintain balance. To work different angles, vary the angle of your feet from straight ahead to slightly outward to inward.

Once you have your balance, slowly lift your heels as high as you can (figure 7.6b). Exhale as you ascend. Pause briefly at the top of the movement.

Slowly lower your heels, going past the starting position to a gentle stretch (figure 7.6c). You should feel no pain in your calves, only a stretch. Maintain an upright position with your knees straight. Inhale as you lower your heels.

Figure 7.6   *Standing Heel Raise (Free Weight)

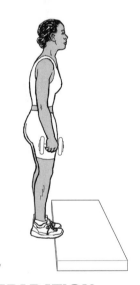

a

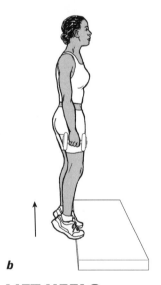

b

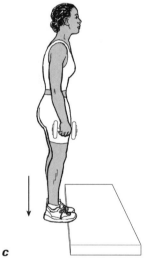

c

PREPARATION

1. Find an elevated, stable surface approximately 6 inches (15 centimeters) high
2. Hold a dumbbell in each hand
3. Place feet hip-width apart
4. Place balls of both feet near edge of platform
5. Lean forward keeping torso erect and knees straight

LIFT HEELS

1. Slowly raise heels as high as possible
2. Pause momentarily at top of movement
3. Exhale as you ascend

LOWER

1. Slowly lower heels to full stretch (no pain)
2. Do not move torso or flex knees
3. Inhale as you descend

Misstep

Your knees flex and extend during the movement.

Correction

Keep your knees straight—but not locked—throughout the exercise.

Misstep

You don't lower your heels to a full stretch.

Correction

Allow the heels to drop down below the platform to the point at which you feel a stretch. Do not go too far; you shouldn't feel pain or discomfort.

Leg Drill 1.   *Choose One Exercise*

After reading about the characteristics and techniques of the exercises and the type of equipment required for each, you are ready to put what you have learned to use. Consider the availability of equipment and access to spotters in your situation, then select one of the following exercises to use in your program:

- Lunge (free weight)
- Leg press (multi- or single-unit weight machine)

Write your leg exercise choice on the workout chart in the "Exercise" column (see page 126). If you intend to include the machine *knee extension or *knee curl or the free-weight *back squat or *standing heel raise, record it on the workout chart immediately after the leg exercise selected above.

Success Check

- Consider availability of equipment.
- Consider need for a spotter and the availability of qualified people.
- Consider time available.
- Choose a leg exercise and record it on the workout chart.

Leg Drill 2.   *Warm-Up and Trial Loads for Basic Exercises*

This practice procedure answers the question "How much weight or load should I use?" Using the coefficient associated with the leg exercise you selected and the formula shown in figure 7.7, determine the trial load. (See step 2, pages 18-20, for more information on using this formula.) Round off your results to the closest 5-pound (2.25-kilogram) increment or to the closest weight-stack plate. For the lunge exercise, divide the loads you calculated by two to equal the weight of each individual dumbbell. Use one-half of the amount determined for the trial load for your warm-up load in the exercise. These loads will be used in drills 4 and 5.

Success Check

- Determine your trial load by multiplying your body weight by the correct coefficient.
- Determine your warm-up load by dividing your trial load by two.
- Round off your trial and warm-up loads to the nearest 5-pound increment or to the closest weight-stack plate.
- Write down your warm-up and trial loads.

Calculations of Warm-Up and Trial Loads for Leg Exercises

Body weight	(Exercise)		Coefficient		Trial load	Warm-up load
		Female				
BWT = _____	(FW–lunge)	×	.10	=	_____	_____
BWT = _____	(C–leg press)	×	1.00	=	_____	_____
		Male				
BWT = _____	(FW–lunge)	×	.10	=	_____	_____
BWT = _____	(C–leg press)	×	1.30	=	_____	_____

BWT = body weight, FW = free weight, C = cam, M = multi- or single-unit machine exercise.

Note: If you are a male who weighs more than 175 lbs. (79 kg), record your body weight as 175 (79). If you are a female who weighs more than 140 lbs. (63.5 kg), record your body weight as 140 (63.5).

Figure 7.7 Warm-up and trial load determination for basic leg exercises.

Leg Drill 3. *Determine Trial Load for *Knee Extension, *Knee Curl, *Back Squat, and *Standing Heel Raise*

If you are an experienced lifter who has decided to add the *knee extension, *knee curl, *back squat, or *standing heel raise, follow the directions to determine your trial load. (See step 2, pages 18-20, for more information.)

Based on your previous experience and knowledge of the weight that you can lift, select a weight that will allow you to perform 12 to 15 reps. Calculate the warm-up load by multiplying the trial load by .6, and round off the number to the nearest 5-pound increment (figure 7.8). For the *standing heel raise, divide the loads you cal-

culated by two to determine the weight of each dumbbell. These loads will be used in drill 4.

Success Check

- Select a weight that will allow 12 to 15 reps.
- Determine the warm-up load by multiplying the trial load by .6.
- Round off the warm-up load to the nearest 5-pound increment or to the closest weight-stack plate.
- Write down your warm-up and trial loads.

Calculation of Warm-Up Load for Additional Exercise

Exercise	Estimated trial load for 12-15 reps				Warm-up load
*Knee extension	_____	×	.6	=	_____
*Knee curl	_____	×	.6	=	_____
*Back squat	_____	×	.6	=	_____
*Standing heel raise	_____	×	.6	=	_____

Figure 7.8 Formula for determining the warm-up load for the *knee extension, *knee curl, *back squat, or *standing heel raise.

Leg Drill 4. *Practice Proper Technique*

In this procedure, you are to perform 15 reps with the warm-up load determined in drill 2 (lunge or leg press) or drill 3 (*knee extension, *knee curl, *back squat, or *standing heel raise). If you are an experienced lifter who has decided to add the *back squat, practice it first. If you decided to add the *knee extension, *knee curl, or *standing heel raise exercise, practice it last.

Review the illustrations and instructions for the exercise, focusing on proper grip and body positioning. Visualize the movement pattern through the full range of motion. Inhale when you are ready to execute the exercise, then perform the movement with a slow, controlled velocity, remembering to exhale through the sticking point. Ask a qualified lifter to observe and assess your technique.

If you selected the free-weight *back squat, you need a spotter. You also need to practice the skills of spotting this exercise. Identify a spotter with whom you will take turns completing the drill.

Instead of performing 15 reps in a continuous manner, practice racking the bar after each repetition. Alternate responsibilities so that you and your partner both have a chance to develop the techniques that are required in performing and spotting this exercise. Ask a qualified person to observe and assess your performance in the basic techniques.

Success Check

- For the *back squat, all rackings are performed correctly.
- For all exercises, movement pattern, velocity, and breathing are correct.

Leg Drill 5. *Determine Training Load*

This practice procedure will help you determine an appropriate training load designed to produce 12 to 15 reps. If you selected the leg press, perform as many reps as possible with the calculated trial load from drill 2. Make sure that you execute the reps correctly.

If you selected the lunge, do not perform a maximal number of reps because you will have extraordinarily sore muscles for the next several days. Instead, over the course of multiple weeks of consistent training, gradually increase the weight of the dumbbells until the 12- to 15-rep range is achieved.

If you executed 12 to 15 reps with the trial load, then your trial load is your training load. Record this number as your training load for this exercise on the workout chart (see page 100). If you did not perform 12 to 15 reps, go to drill 6 to make adjustments to the load.

Success Check

- Check for correct load.
- Maintain proper and safe technique during each rep.

Leg Drill 6. *Make Needed Load Adjustments*

If you performed fewer than 12 reps with your trial load, the load is too heavy and you need to lighten it. On the other hand, if you performed more than 15 reps, the load is too light and you need to increase it. Use table 7.1 to determine the adjustment you need to make. Figure 7.9 shows the formula for making load adjustments.

Table 7.1 Load Adjustments

Reps completed	Adjustments (lbs.)
<7	–15
8-9	–10
10-11	–5
16-17	+5
18-19	+10
>20	+15

Adjustments of Training Load		
Trial load	Adjustment	Training load
_____ +	_____ =	_____

Figure 7.9 Making adjustments to the training load for leg exercises.

Success Check

- Check correct use of load adjustment chart (table 7.1).
- Record your training load on the workout chart (see page 126).

SUCCESS SUMMARY FOR LEG EXERCISES

This step involved selecting one leg exercise for which you have the needed equipment, and perhaps one or two more if you have already been training. Using a proper grip; the correct body position, movement, and breathing patterns; and accurate warm-up and training loads will ensure a positive outcome.

Before Taking the Next Step

Honestly answer each of the following questions. If you answer yes to all of the questions relevant to your level and exercise selection, you are ready to move on to step 8.

1. Have you selected a basic leg exercise? If you are an advanced lifter, do you want to add the *knee extension, *knee curl, *back squat, or *standing heel raise?
2. Have you recorded your exercise selection(s) on the workout chart?
3. Have you determined warm-up and training loads for the exercise(s) you selected?
4. Have you recorded the warm-up and training loads on the workout chart?
5. Have you learned the proper technique for performing the exercise(s) you selected?
6. If an exercise you selected requires a spotter, have you identified a qualified person? Have you learned the proper spotting techniques?

Once you have determined your training load(s) and recorded it in your workout chart, you are ready to move on to step 8, in which you will select exercises that will develop the abdominal muscles. The exercises include the bent-knee sit-up, the machine trunk curl, and the *twisting trunk curl.

Abdominal Exercises

The abdominal muscles are the major supporting muscles for the front of the torso. They not only support and protect internal organs but also aid the muscles of the low back to align and support the spine for good posture and lifting activities.

Properly developed abdominal muscles serve as a biological girdle to flatten your waistline. Although there is no such thing as spot reducing (fat reduction in only one area), strong abdominal muscles make the area smaller and look tighter even though the fat may still be there.

The abdominal muscles include the rectus abdominis, which causes the trunk to bend or flex forward, and the obliques, which assist the rectus abdominis and cause trunk rotation and bending to the side.

The exercises in this step are the bent-knee sit-up, the machine abdominal curl, and the *twisting trunk curl. The straight-leg (knees straight) sit-up is not included here because it relies heavily on the hip-flexor muscles (especially the iliopsoas) and does not effectively train the abdominal muscles. Plus, it may contribute to low back problems.

The bent-knee sit-up and the *twisting trunk curl are no-weight exercises. All you need for these exercises is your own body. If you have access to a cam machine, you may select the trunk curl to develop your abdominal muscles. These machines come in various designs, so be sure to follow the signs or ask for assistance if the directions in this step do not match the machine in your facility.

BENT-KNEE SIT-UP

Prepare for this exercise by lying down on your back with your head, back, and feet flat on a mat (figure 8.1a). In this position, your knees will be flexed 90 to 110 degrees. Fold your arms across your chest with your hands on opposite shoulders.

Begin the upward execution as you inhale and pull your chin to your chest. Then contract your abdominal muscles to lift your torso until your shoulders are elevated 30 degrees (figure 8.1b). Do not go past 30 degrees (a position in which only your shoulders are off the floor).

Be sure to exhale when nearing the point of greatest flexion (upward position). This movement should be slow and controlled; do not use momentum created by lurching forward with the head, arms, and shoulders. Pause briefly at the top point.

The downward execution follows the pause at the top. Inhale as you lower (figure 8.1c). Be sure to keep your chin on your chest until your shoulders touch the floor. Then allow your head to touch. Make this part of the exercise slow and controlled by keeping your abdominal muscles contracted; you will receive equal benefit from both the upward and downward phases. Your low back, buttocks, and feet should remain in contact with the floor throughout the exercise.

Misstep

Your shoulders lower rapidly, followed by a bouncing action upward.

Correction

Slowly return your upper back, shoulders, and head to the starting position. Pause on the floor before beginning the next rep.

A higher number of reps (15 to 25) is encouraged to promote tone and muscular endurance. However, you should not sacrifice quality for quantity. Be sure to perform at least 15 reps, even it means that you need to rest during the set.

If you find that this exercise is too easy after you have performed it for a period of time, increase the difficulty by placing your hands behind your head or by lightly touching your ears to give the added weight of your arms. Never pull your head upward, because this action could cause soreness or injury to your neck muscles.

Figure 8.1   Bent-Knee Sit-Up

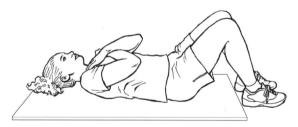

a

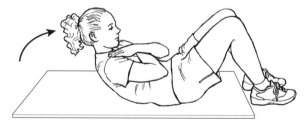

b

PREPARATION

1. Lie down with back flat on floor
2. Flex knees at 90 to 110 degrees
3. Place feet flat on floor
4. Fold arms across chest

LIFT

1. Curl chin to chest first
2. Raise shoulders and upper back to 30 degrees
3. Pause
4. Exhale during upward phase

LOWER

1. Slowly return to starting position
2. Keep chin to chest until shoulders touch floor
3. Lower head to floor
4. Pause, do not bounce, at bottom
5. Inhale during downward phase

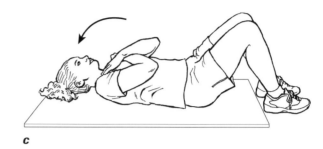

c

Misstep

Your buttocks lift off the floor just prior to upward movement.

Correction

Start the exercise with your head, shoulders, upper back, and low back in contact with the floor. Keep your low back and buttocks in contact with the floor throughout each rep.

Misstep

You use momentum to complete the movement.

Correction

Concentrate on using your abdominal muscles only to complete the movement. Using momentum won't give you toned abs.

Most errors associated with the bent-knee sit-up involve speed. You will have a tendency to lurch forward and then quickly fall back to the starting position. Keep the movements slow and controlled in both the upward and downward movement phases.

TRUNK CURL

Assume an erect sitting position in the cam machine, with your shoulders and upper arms firmly against the pads. Adjust the height of the seat so that the axis of rotation is level with the lower part of your sternum (midchest). Place your ankles behind the roller pad, with your knees spread and your hands crossing in front of you (figure 8.2a).

While maintaining this position, shorten the distance between your rib cage and navel by contracting your abdominal muscles only (figure 8.2b). Pause in the fully contracted position, then return slowly to the starting position (figure 8.2c). Exhale during contraction and inhale during relaxation.

| Figure 8.2 | **Trunk Curl (Cam Machine)** |

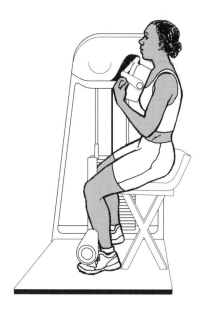

a

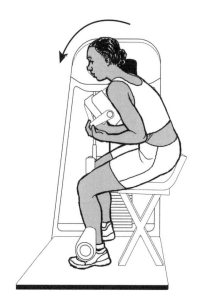

b

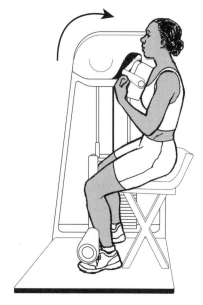

c

PREPARATION

1. Sit erect with shoulders and upper arms firmly against pads
2. Adjust seat so axis of rotation is level with lower part of sternum
3. Place ankles behind roller pads
4. Spread knees
5. Cross arms

CURL

1. Shorten distance between rib cage and navel by contracting abdominal muscles only
2. Keep legs relaxed as chest moves down and forward
3. Exhale during contraction
4. Pause in contracted position

RETURN

1. Return slowly to starting position
2. Inhale while returning to starting position

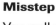

Misstep

You pull with your hands and shoulders.

Correction

Concentrate on contracting your abdominal muscles only.

Misstep

Your shoulders and upper arms come off the pads.

Correction

Think, "Shoulders and upper arms stay firmly against the pads throughout the exercise."

*TWISTING TRUNK CURL

If you are an experienced lifter who is ready for a second abdominal exercise, consider adding the *twisting trunk curl. This exercise is similar to the bent-knee sit-up in that it trains the same muscle group with nearly the same movement pattern. The two main differences are that you place your feet on a bench or chair with your hips and knees at 90-degree angles and you alternately curl your shoulders toward the *opposite* knee (the twisting motion) during the upward phase.

Prepare by lying on your back and propping your feet on a chair or weight bench (figure 8.3a). Your knees and hips should be at 90-degree angles. Fold your arms across your chest.

Inhale and curl your chin to your chest. Contract your abdominal muscles and slowly lift your shoulders off the floor. Twist your torso so that your right shoulder goes toward your left knee (figure 8.3b). Exhale when you near the highest position and pause at the top of the movement.

Slowly return to the starting position, using your abdominal muscles to control your body on the way down (figure 8.3c). Keep your chin to your chest until your shoulders touch the floor. Inhale as you lower to the floor.

On the next repetition, twist your torso so that your left shoulder goes toward your right knee. Continue, alternating the direction in which you twist with each repetition.

| Figure 8.3 | *Twisting Trunk Curl |

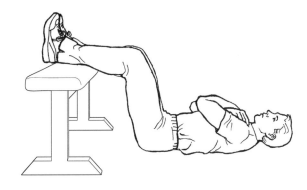

a

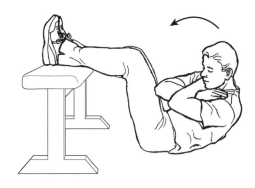

b

PREPARATION

1. Lie down with back flat on floor
2. Place feet on bench or chair
3. Fold arms across chest
4. Inhale

CURL

1. Curl chin to chest first
2. Alternately curl shoulders and upper back toward opposite knee
3. Exhale when nearing highest position
4. Pause

(continued)

Figure 8.3 (continued)

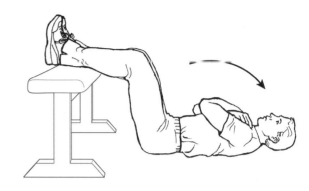

LOWER

1. Return slowly to starting position
2. Keep chin to chest until shoulders touch floor
3. Inhale during downward movement

c

Misstep

Your buttocks lift off the floor just prior to the upward movement.

Correction

Start the exercise with your head, shoulders, upper back, and low back in contact with the floor. Keep your low back and buttocks in contact with the floor throughout each rep.

Misstep

You use momentum to complete the movement.

Correction

Concentrate on using your abdominal muscles only to complete the movement. Using momentum won't give you toned abs.

Most errors associated with the *twisting trunk curl involve speed. You will have a tendency to lurch forward and then quickly fall back to the starting position. Keep the movements slow and controlled in both the upward and downward phases. Slowly lower your upper back, shoulders, and head to the starting position. Pause on the floor before beginning the next repetition.

Abdominal Drill 1. *Choose One Exercise*

After reading about the characteristics and techniques of the exercises and the type of equipment required for each, you are ready to put what you have learned to use. Consider what equipment is available to you, then select one of the following exercises to use in your program:

- Bent-knee sit-up
- Trunk curl (cam machine)

Write your abdominal exercise choice on the workout chart in the "Exercise" column (see page 126). If you intend to include the *twisting trunk curl, record it on the workout chart immediately after the abdominal exercise previously selected. Because you will not be using any additional weight, simply record the number of repetitions and leave the space for the load blank.

Success Check

- Consider availability of equipment.
- Consider time available.
- Choose an abdominal exercise and record it on the workout chart.

Abdominal Drill 2. *Warm-Up and Trial Loads for Trunk Curl*

This practice procedure will answer the question "How much weight or load should I use?" If you chose the bent-knee sit-up or the *twisting trunk curl, you will not need to establish warm-up, trial, and training loads. Continue to drill 3 and ignore comments concerning warm-up and training loads. If you chose the machine trunk curl, continue with the following procedures.

For the trunk curl (cam machine) exercise, use the formula shown in figure 8.4 to determine the trial load. (See step 2, pages 18-20, for more information on using this formula.) Round your results to the closest weight-stack plate. Use one-half of the amount determined for the trial load for your warm-up load in the exercise. These loads will be used in drills 3 and 4.

Success Check

- Determine your trial load for the trunk curl by multiplying your body weight by the correct coefficient.
- Determine your warm-up load by dividing your trial load by two.
- Round off your trial and warm-up loads to the closest weight-stack plate.
- Write down your warm-up and trial loads.

Calculations of Warm-Up and Trial Loads for Trunk Curl

Body weight	(Exercise)	Coefficient	Trial load	Warm-up load
		Female		
BWT = _____	(C–trunk curl)	× .20 =	_____	_____
		Male		
BWT = _____	(C–trunk curl)	× .20 =	_____	_____

BWT = body weight, FW = free weight, C = cam, M = multi- or single-unit machine exercise.

Note: If you are a male who weighs more than 175 lbs. (79 kg), record your body weight as 175 (79). If you are a female who weighs more than 140 lbs. (63.5 kg), record your body weight as 140 (63.5).

Figure 8.4 Warm-up and trial load determination for trunk curl.

Abdominal Drill 3. *Practice Proper Technique*

In this procedure, you are to perform 15 reps of the exercise you have chosen. If you chose the trunk curl, use the warm-up load determined in drill 2. If you are an experienced lifter who has decided to add the *twisting trunk curl, practice it last.

Review the illustrations and instructions for proper body positioning. Visualize the movement pattern through the full range of motion. Inhale when you are ready to execute the exercise, then perform the movement with a slow, controlled velocity, remembering to exhale through the sticking point. Ask a qualified lifter to observe and assess your technique.

Success Check

- Check movement pattern.
- Check velocity of movements.
- Check breathing.

Abdominal Drill 4. *Determine Training Load for Trunk Curl*

If you chose the bent-knee sit-up or *twisting trunk curl, you do not need to determine warm-up, trial, or training loads. Skip drills 4 and 5 and proceed to the success summary.

This practice procedure will help you determine an appropriate training load, designed to produce 12 to 15 reps, for the trunk curl. Use the calculated trial load from drill 2 and perform as many reps as possible with this load. Make sure that you execute the reps correctly.

CAUTION **For this exercise, do not perform more than 25 repetitions even if you are able to do so.**

If you executed 12 to 15 reps with the trial load, then your trial load is your training load. Record this number as your training load for this exercise on the workout chart (see page 126). If you did not perform 12 to 15 reps, go to drill 5 to make adjustments to the load.

Success Check

- Check for correct load.
- Maintain proper and safe technique during each rep.

Abdominal Drill 5. *Make Needed Load Adjustments for Trunk Curl*

If you performed fewer than 12 reps with your trial load, the load is too heavy and you need to lighten it. On the other hand, if you performed more than 15 reps, the load is too light and you need to increase it. Use table 8.1 to determine the adjustment you need to make. Figure 8.5 shows the formula for making load adjustments.

Success Check

- Check correct use of load-adjustment chart (table 8.1).
- Record your training load on the workout chart (see page 126).

Table 8.1 Load Adjustments

Reps completed	Adjustments (lbs.)
<7	−15
8-9	−10
10-11	−5
16-17	+5
18-19	+10
>20	+15

Adjustments of Training Load

Trial load	Adjustment	Training load
_____ +	_____ =	_____

Figure 8.5 Making adjustments to the training load for the trunk curl.

SUCCESS SUMMARY FOR ABDOMINAL EXERCISES

In this step, you learned how to perform three exercises that can be used to strengthen and flatten the abdominal area. Regardless of which exercise you selected, be sure to perform it in a slow, controlled manner and complete 15 to 25 repetitions during each workout, depending on the abdominal exercise selected.

Before Taking the Next Step

Honestly answer each of the following questions. If you answer yes to all of the questions relevant to your level and exercise selection, you are ready to move on to step 9.

1. Have you selected a basic abdominal exercise? If you are an advanced lifter, do you want to add the *twisting trunk curl?
2. Have you recorded your exercise selection on the workout chart?
3. If you chose the trunk curl, have you determined warm-up and training loads?
4. Did you record your warm-up and training loads on the workout chart?
5. Have you learned the proper technique for performing the exercise(s) you selected?

Once you have determined your training load and recorded it on your workout chart, you are ready to move on to step 9, in which you will select total-body exercises for your program. You may select from two exercises: the hang clean and the push press. Both of these involve the use of a barbell and each requires a higher level of muscular coordination than any of the exercises included in steps 3 through 8. If you are new to weight training, you will want to wait a couple of months before adding these exercises to your workouts. If you are experienced, adding one or both of them to your workout will provide you with a more well-rounded and challenging program.

Total-Body Exercises

In this step, you have an opportunity to add a total-body exercise—the hang clean or the push press—to your basic program. Total-body exercises train major muscles of the upper and lower body at the same time. These exercises involve quick movements of the barbell and are especially popular among athletes because they develop total-body strength. Performing barbell exercises in less time (also called *power*) improves performance in sports that have an explosive or speed–strength component.

Total-body exercises involve many muscle groups. A high level of muscular coordination is required to perform them correctly. Thus, if you are just beginning a weight training program, the total-body exercises included in this step are not appropriate for you. To give you time to practice and gain experience in weight training in general, it is best to wait at least six weeks before adding one of these exercises.

If you choose to include a full-body exercise, perform it first during your workout. Because these exercises involve many muscle groups

and require a high level of muscular coordination for correct technique, you need your muscles to be as fresh as possible. By performing them first, you can give attention to proper technique while you are least fatigued.

Unlike other steps, all of these exercises use free weights only, so you will need access to a bar, weight plates, and two locks. Also, because the exercises are performed quickly and require extra attention to proper technique, they must be performed in an area away from others who are training. The area should have some floor protection in case you drop the bar quickly.

A spotter should not be used in these exercises because if something goes wrong, a spotter attempting to help or catch the bar could easily be injured or could cause injury to you. Do not ask someone to spot you in these exercises. If you experience balance or execution problems while performing them, simply allow the bar to drop while you back away from its downward path.

HANG CLEAN

In the hang clean exercise, the bar moves from the thighs to the shoulders in one quick, powerful jumping movement. Initially the bar is on the thighs, just above the knees, not on the floor. The upward phase requires a forceful, rapid extension of the hips, knees, and ankles followed by shrugging the shoulders and pulling with the arms to lift the bar to the front of the shoulders.

Begin this exercise with the bar at a midthigh (hang) position (figure 9.1*a*). The techniques used to reach the midthigh position are the same as the preparation and upward execution (floor-to-thigh) phases described in step 1 (see figure 1.5, page 6, and figure 1.7, page 7).

From this starting position, rapidly jump straight up (figure 9.1*b*). Completely extend the knees and hips. Think about jumping up, pushing through the floor, and fully lengthening your lower body. Immediately follow the jump with a strong shoulder-shrugging motion (figure 9.1*c*). Up to this point your arms have functioned like ropes that attach the bar to your shoulders (your elbows have been straight) to pull the bar upward. However, at the end of the shrugging motion, your elbows flex, moving up and to the side, to continue pulling the bar as high as possible.

Misstep

The bar swings away from your thighs and hips.

Correction

Concentrate on pulling the bar straight up and keeping it close to your thighs and hips.

Once the bar reaches its highest point (figure 9.1*d*), quickly shift your body under it to catch the weight while rapidly rotating your elbows down and under and then up in front of the bar as it touches your shoulders and clavicle (figure 9.1*e*). Do not let your elbows flex too soon; wait to do so until the shrug is at its highest point. As your elbows rotate around the bar, flex your knees and catch the barbell on the front of your shoulders. At the same time, your knees should act like shock absorbers to smoothly cushion the downward momentum. Never catch the weight with your knees fully extended because doing so could injure your

back. Move your upper arms parallel to the floor and, after gaining a balanced position, finish the exercise by standing erect. Exhale as the bar lands on your shoulders.

To return the bar to the midthigh (hang) position, slowly and with control unrack the bar and allow it to descend until it reaches your thighs (figure 9.1*f*). Simultaneously, flex your hips and knees to reduce the impact on your thighs. Your back should remain straight with your shoulders pulled back and the bar close to your chest and abdominal area. After the last rep of the set, squat to lower the bar past your knees and onto the floor.

Figure 9.1   **Hang Clean**

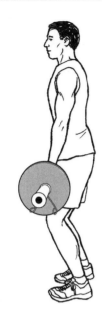

a

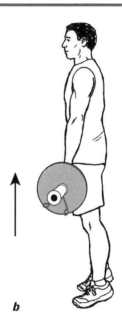

b

PREPARATION

1. Properly lift bar from floor to thighs
2. Start exercise from midthigh position

JUMP

1. Jump up explosively
2. Keep bar close to body as hips drive forward
3. Keep elbows straight
4. Fully extend (straighten) knees and hips

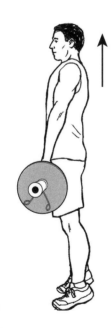

c

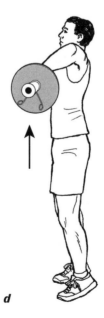

d

SHRUG

1. Rapidly shrug the shoulders
2. Shrug as high as possible
3. Keep elbows straight

HIGHEST BAR HEIGHT

1. Flex elbows and move them up and to side
2. Keep elbows above wrists
3. Continue pulling bar as high as possible

(continued)

Figure 9.1 *(continued)*

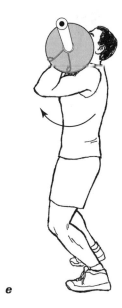

e

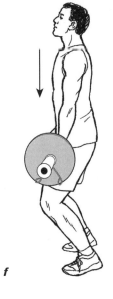

f

CATCH

1. Rotate elbows down under, then up in front of bar
2. Catch bar (rack it) on front of shoulders
3. Flex knees and hips to absorb bar's impact
4. Exhale
5. Move upper arms to be parallel to floor
6. Gain balance and stand up straight

UNRACK

1. Unrack bar
2. Flex knees and hips
3. Allow bar to lower to thighs
4. Keep shoulders back and back flat
5. Keep bar close to chest and abdomen
6. After final repetition, allow bar to lower past knees
7. Squat to set bar on floor
8. Keep bar close to thighs, knees, and shins

Misstep

You rely on your arms to accelerate the bar off your thighs.

Correction

Do not think about your arms doing active work until you have jumped up.

Misstep

Your knees are straight when you catch the bar.

Correction

Concentrate on flexing your knees, which provides give to your shoulders as you rack the bar on them and dissipates much of the impact.

Because of the complexity of this exercise, you may perform multiple errors in one rep or develop technique flaws. Be diligent about perfecting your technique with this or any total-body exercise. Many of the common errors and corrections seen with this exercise are similar to those described in the "Lifting the Bar Off the Floor" section of step 1 (see page 5).

PUSH PRESS

In the push press, the bar moves from the shoulders to overhead in one quick and powerful jumping movement, similar to the hang clean. For this exercise, begin with the bar where it ends during the hang clean—at the front of the shoulders. The upward phase resembles the standing press (see figure 5.1, page 56), but the push press requires a forceful, rapid extension of the hips, knees, and ankles, followed by a pushing motion of the arms to lift the bar to a stable position over the head with the elbows fully extended. Exhalation occurs as the bar is returned to the shoulders between each repetition.

You will need to use the techniques you learned in step 1 (see figure 1.5, page 6; figure 1.7, page 7; and figure 1.8, page 9) and in the hang clean exercise (figure 9.1) to properly lift the bar off the floor up to the shoulders before you can actually begin the push press exercise. Alternatively, you can lift the bar out of a squat rack with supports already positioned at shoulder level.

The bar should be resting on your shoulders, clavicles (collarbones), and hands (figure 9.2a). From this starting position, flex the hips and knees at a slow to moderate speed to move the bar in a straight path downward (figure 9.2b). This downward movement is not a full squat but rather a dip to a depth not to exceed the catch position of the hang clean. Do not lean forward or backward as you dip. Keep your torso erect and your head in a neutral position, and do not change the position of your arms.

Immediately after reaching the lowest position of the dip, reverse the movement by rap-idly extending your hips, knees, and ankles. Be sure to fully extend your knees and hips during the drive. Think about jumping up, pushing through the floor, and fully lengthening your lower body. As your lower-body joints reach full extension, slightly tip your head backward to allow the bar to pass by your chin (or else it will hit you). At this point you begin pushing upward with your arms (figure 9.2c). To be sure that the bar travels straight up, be sure to "jump" straight up with your torso erect.

Catch the bar directly overhead with fully extended elbows and your hips and knees flexed to absorb the weight. Having your knees flexed provides give as you rack the bar on your shoulders, dissipating much of the impact. Your torso should be erect with your head in a neutral position directly under the bar, with your eyes focused forward (figure 9.2d). To keep your torso from leaning back when you catch the bar, think, "Torso, head, and bar form a straight line." Once the bar is balanced overhead, stand up to a fully erect position by extending your hips and knees.

To return the bar to the beginning position, slowly and with control allow it to descend until it reaches your shoulders (figure 9.2e). Exhale as the bar reaches your shoulders and simultaneously flex your hips and knees to reduce the impact. Your back should remain straight with your shoulders pulled back and your chest held up and out. After the last rep of the set, lower the bar to your thighs, then squat to set it on the floor.

Figure 9.2   Push Press

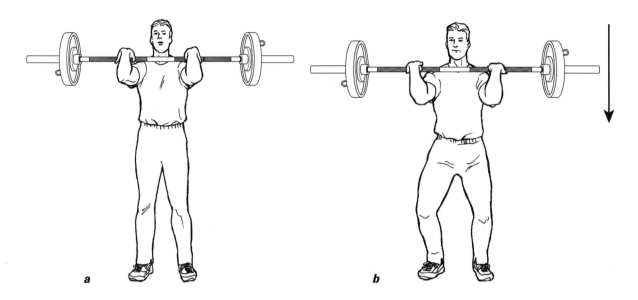

a

b

PREPARATION

1. Properly lift bar from floor to thighs
2. Properly lift bar from thighs to shoulders
3. Start exercise with bar at front of shoulders

DIP

1. Flex hips and knees at a slow to moderate speed
2. Move bar downward in straight path
3. Keep torso erect and head in neutral position
4. Do not change position of arms

DRIVE

1. Jump up explosively
2. Tip head back slightly
3. Extend (straighten) knees and hips fully
4. Push up with arms
5. Keep eyes focused forward

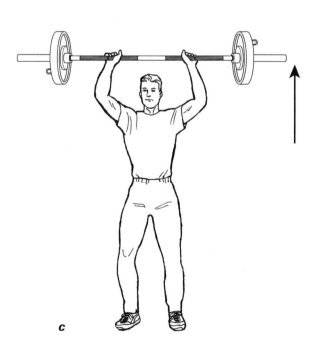

c

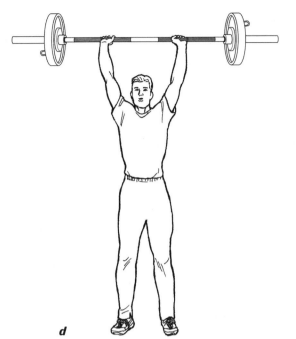

d

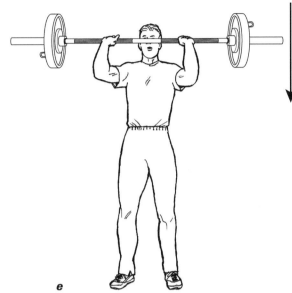

e

CATCH

1. Catch bar directly overhead with fully extended elbows
2. Flex knees and hips to absorb bar's impact
3. Keep torso erect and eyes focused forward
4. Gain balance, then stand up straight

LOWER

1. Allow bar to lower to shoulders
2. Exhale as bar reaches shoulders
3. Flex knees and hips
4. Keep shoulders back and back flat
5. After final repetition, unrack bar from shoulders
6. Allow bar to lower to thighs
7. Keep bar close to chest and abdomen
8. Allow bar to lower past knees
9. Squat to set bar on floor
10. Keep bar close to thighs, knees, and shins

Misstep

Your arms extend unevenly.

Correction

Keep both of your arms extending in unison by visually focusing and concentrating on the arm that lags behind.

Misstep

The bar is behind or slightly ahead of your head in the catch position.

Correction

Catch the bar directly over the head with fully extended elbows, an erect torso, and the head in a neutral position.

Like the hang clean, this exercise can be a challenge to learn and master. You may perform several technique mistakes at one time.

Common errors and corrections are similar to those described for the hang clean and the standing press (see step 5, page 56).

Total-Body Drill 1.   *Choose One Exercise*

After reading about the characteristics and techniques of these two total-body exercises and the type of equipment they require, you are ready to put this information to use. Consider the availability of equipment and your situation, then select one of the following exercises to use in your program:

- Hang clean
- Push press

Write your total-body exercise choice on the workout chart in the "Exercise" column (see page 126).

Performing any total-body exercise first in your workout is critically important (regardless of where you wrote the exercise name on your workout chart). Total-body exercises involve many muscle groups, and performing them correctly requires a high level of muscular coordination. As a result, you must perform them before other exercises so that you can give attention to proper technique while you are least fatigued.

Success Check

- Consider availability of equipment.
- Consider availability of a designated area away from other lifters.
- Consider time available.
- Choose a full-body exercise and record it on the workout chart.

Total-Body Drill 2.   *Warm-Up and Trial Loads for Full-Body Exercises*

This practice procedure answers the question "How much weight or load should I use?" If you are an experienced lifter who is ready to add a total-body exercise, follow the directions to determine the trial load.

In steps 3 through 8, you determined trial and warm-up loads that would allow you to perform 12 to 15 reps. Because total-body exercises involve multiple large and small muscle groups of the upper and lower body and require a high level of skill to perform correctly, they can cause fatigue very quickly. In that tired state, even a well-trained lifter will not be able to repeatedly perform explosive, quick movements; as a result, the quality of the exercise can severely decrease. Total-body exercises that are performed too slowly, with too much weight, or for too many

reps lose much of their effectiveness. Therefore, for your warm-up, trial, and even your workout sets, limit the number of reps to 6 to 8 for the hang clean and the push press.

The most accurate way to determine trial and warm-up loads for total-body exercises requires you to have previously performed the hang clean or the push press to give you an idea of how much load you can handle and still produce explosive, quick reps.

If a total-body exercise is new to you, go back to step 5 and determine warm-up and trial loads for the standing press (see page 56). If you did not select the standing press as your shoulder exercise from step 5, go back and read the technique points that accompany figure 5.1. Complete shoulder drill 2 for the standing press and write down the trial load. When doing the hang clean or the push press perform only 6-8 reps with the warm-up load—not 12-15 reps. That way you can be sure that you will be able to perform the exercises powerfully and with good technique without excessive fatigue. Use the formula shown in figure 9.3 to determine the warm-up load.

Success Check

- Determine a trial load based on shoulder drill 2 for the standing press (see step 5).
- Determine the warm-up load by multiplying the trial load by .6.
- Round off the warm-up load to the nearest 5-pound (2.25-kilogram) increment.
- Write down your warm-up and trial loads.

Calculation of Warm-Up Loads for Total-Body Exercises

Exercise	Estimated trial load				Warm-up load
Hang clean	_____	×	.6	=	_____
Push press	_____	×	.6	=	_____

Figure 9.3 Formula for determining the warm-up load for the hang clean or the push press. The estimated trial load is the same as the load determined for the standing press in step 5.

Total-Body Drill 3. *Practice Proper Technique*

In this procedure, you are to perform 6 to 8 reps with the warm-up load determined in drill 2. Be sure you practice the total-body exercise *before* any other exercise.

Review the illustrations and instructions for the exercise. Visualize the movement pattern through the full range of motion. Asking a qualified person to observe and assess your technique is especially important for a total-body exercise.

Success Check

- Check movement pattern.
- Check velocity.
- Check breathing.

Total-Body Drill 4. *Determine Training Load*

Now go back to shoulder drill 5 of step 5 and use the trial load of the standing press to determine the training load for that exercise.

Add 10 pounds to the standing press and this load becomes the training load you should use for the hang clean or the push press. Record this number as your training load for your selected total-body exercise on the workout chart, and skip total-body drill 5. Remember that the high-est repetition range for a total-body exercise is 6 to 8 per set.

If you did not perform 6 to 8 reps, continue to total-body drill 5.

Success Check

- Check for correct load.
- Maintain proper and safe technique during each rep.

Total-Body Drill 5.   *Make Needed Load Adjustments*

If you performed fewer than 6 reps with your trial load, the load is too heavy and you should lighten it. On the other hand, If you performed more than 8 reps, the load is too light and you need to increase it. Use table 9.1 that has been modified for the total body exercises to determine the adjustment you need to make. Figure 9.4 shows the formula for making load adjustments. The resulting load is what you will use for the hang clean or the push press exercise. Again, keep in mind that the highest repetition range for a total-body exercise is 6 to 8 per set.

Success Check

- Check correct use of load-adjustment chart (table 9.1).
- Record your training load on the workout chart (see page 126).

Table 9.1   Load Adjustments

Reps completed	Adjustments (lbs.)
1	−15
2-3	−10
4-5	−5
9-10	+5
11-12	+10
> 12	+15

Adjustments of Training Load		
Trial load	Adjustment	Training load
_____	+ _____	= _____

Figure 9.4   Making adjustments to the training load for total-body exercises.

SUCCESS SUMMARY FOR TOTAL-BODY EXERCISES

If you are new to training you may have elected to wait until you are more experienced before adding the hang clean or push press to your workout. If you are more experienced and have added one or both of these exercises, you have taken your program to the next level. Using a proper grip, the correct body position, movement, and breathing patterns, and accurate warm-up and training loads will ensure a positive outcome.

Once you have determined your training load for one or both total-body exercises and recorded it on your workout chart, you are ready to move on to step 10. This step provides instruction on how to approach your first workout now that you have selected all of the exercises for your program.

Before Taking the Next Step

Honestly answer each of the following questions. If you answer yes to all of the questions relevant to your level and exercise selection, you are ready to move on to step 10.

1. Have you selected a total-body exercise?
2. Have you recorded your exercise selection on the workout chart?
3. Have you determined a warm-up and training load for the exercise you selected?
4. Have you recorded the warm-up and training loads on the workout chart?
5. Have you learned the proper technique for performing the exercise you selected?

Training With a Standard Program

Now the fun really begins, because this is when you start training! This step takes you through a series of tasks that are necessary to complete your first workout and to make appropriate changes in the ones that follow. Each workout should contain three parts: a proper warm-up, at least one exercise for each of the large muscle groups from steps 3 through 8 (add a total-body exercise from step 9 after you are better trained), and a proper cool-down.

The well-balanced basic program gets you started on a training schedule. You don't have to worry about other exercises to include, in which order to do them, how many reps or sets to do, or when to make load changes—these decisions have already been made for you. You should follow this program for at least six weeks before tailoring it in any way. It is designed to slowly improve your muscular endurance and give your body time to adapt to the new demands being placed on it.

BASIC PROGRAM

By this point you should have filled out much of the information needed for figure 10.1, the workout chart. You should have selected an exercise for each of the muscle groups and determined a training load for each exercise. This is your basic program; in this step, you will use it to begin your journey to muscular fitness.

Make six copies of the workout chart (figure 10.1) to record your basic program results for six weeks. Remember to properly warm up before each workout and cool down afterward.

The drills at the end of this step will help you determine when and how to make needed changes to your workouts.

For maximum benefits, make a commitment to train three times a week, and allow yourself one day of rest between workouts. For example, try a Monday/Wednesday/Friday or a Tuesday/Thursday/Saturday schedule. If you can train only twice a week, allow no more than three days between sessions—a Monday/Thursday, Tuesday/Saturday, or Wednesday/Sunday regime. With consistent training,

Weight training workout chart (three days a week)

	Muscle area	Exercise	Load × sets × reps	Set	Week Day 1	Week Day 2	Week Day 3
1	Total body*			Wt.			
				Reps			
2	Chest			Wt.			
				Reps			
3	Back			Wt.			
				Reps			
4	Shoulders			Wt.			
				Reps			
5	Biceps			Wt.			
				Reps			
6	Triceps			Wt.			
				Reps			
7	Legs			Wt.			
				Reps			
8	Abdomen			Wt.			
				Reps			
9				Wt.			
				Reps			
10				Wt.			
				Reps			
11				Wt.			
				Reps			
12				Wt.			
				Reps			
Body weight							
Date							
Comments							

* For advanced lifters only. See step 9.

From *Weight Training: Steps to Success, Third Edition*, by Thomas R. Baechle and Roger W. Earle, 2006, Champaign, IL: Human Kinetics.

Figure 10.1 Weight training workout chart for a three-days-a-week program.

you will notice that as your muscular fitness improves, so will your ability to recover from the fatigue of each set.

The basic program begins with one set of 12 to 15 reps for the first workout, two sets of 12 to 15 reps for workouts 2 through 4, and three sets of 12 to 15 reps for workouts 5 through 18. The strategy is that the first four workouts will provide an appropriate level of stress to prepare your body for the more strenuous workouts to follow.

Pay attention to the length of the rest periods; try to be consistent between sets and workouts. The recovery time between each set and exercise should be 1 minute until workout 5, when you can consider shortening it to 45 or 30 seconds. Shortening the rest period will not only improve your level of muscular endurance, it also reduces the amount of time needed to complete a workout. The disadvantage is that if you do not give yourself adequate rest, you will not be able to complete the targeted number of reps. The result would be that you do not accomplish what you set out to do—which is to perform more reps of each exercise.

When you are able to perform two or more reps above the intended number (17 or more) in the last set on two consecutive training days (the *two-for-two rule*), it is time to increase the load. If you are unable to perform 12 reps in two consecutive training sessions, you need to decrease the load. Refer to the load-adjustment chart shown in table 10.1 and make appropriate changes to the load. Refer back to table 9.1 in the previos step for making adjustments to the total body exercises.

Keep in mind two very important points while training. First, all reps should be performed with excellent technique—do not sacrifice technique for additional reps. The quality of the technique used to perform each rep is more important than the number of reps performed. Give each rep in each set your best effort, and apply the two-for-two rule to keep the number of reps in each set between 12 and 15.

Table 10.1 Load Adjustments

Reps completed	Adjustments (lbs.)
<7	–15
8-9	–10
10-11	–5
16-17	+5
18-19	+10
>20	+15

*Use table 9.1 for adjusting total body exercises

Charting Your Program Drill 1.   *Workout 1*

For your first workout, perform one set of each exercise in the order listed on your workout chart. If the training loads are correct, you should be able to perform 12 to 15 repetitions in each set; if not, make adjustments as described in practice procedure 5 in step 2 (see pages 21-22). On your workout chart, record the completed number of reps in each set under the heading "Day 1." Figure 10.2 illustrates where to write in loads and reps performed. After completing a set of an exercise, rest approximately 1 minute before starting the next exercise.

If you select any of the additional exercises included in steps 3 through 8, remember to write them on the workout chart immediately after the basic exercise selected for that step. If you include the total-body exercises described in step 9, be sure to perform them first (regardless of where they are written on the workout chart) because they require fresher muscles than the other exercises.

Success Check

- Check to make sure load selection is correct and bars are loaded evenly.
- Secure plates, bars, and selection keys in weight stacks.
- Use proper exercise and, if necessary, spotting techniques.
- Make appropriate load adjustments, if necessary.

Weight training workout chart (three days a week)

Load goes here

Set 1

Number of reps goes here

Workout day

	Muscle area	Exercise	Load × sets × reps	Set	Week ___ Day 1			Day 2	
					1	2	3	1	2
1	Total body*			Wt.					
				Reps					
2	Chest	Bench press	90	Wt.	90				
				Reps	13				
3	Back	Bent-over row	80	Wt.	80				
				Reps	12				
4	Shoulders	Standing press	60	Wt.	60				
				Reps	15				
5	Biceps	Biceps curl	75	Wt.	75				
				Reps	15				
6	Triceps	Triceps push-down	30	Wt.	30				
				Reps	12				
7	Legs	Leg press	165	Wt.	165				
				Reps	15				
8	Abdomen	Trunk curl	—	Wt.	—				
				Reps	20				

Figure 10.2 Recording loads and reps.

Charting Your Program Drill 2. *Workouts 2 Through 4*

If you are training with a partner, arrange your workouts so that you alternate turns performing an exercise until both of you have completed the desired number of sets. For workouts 2 through 4, perform two sets of each of the exercises in the order listed on your workout chart. Again, if the training loads are correct, you should be able to perform 12 to 15 reps in a set (exception; total body exercises). If not, you will need to make adjustments as described in practice procedure 5 in step 2 (see pages 21-22).

After completing a set of an exercise, rest 1 minute before starting the next set. On your workout chart, record the reps and sets you've completed under the proper headings. See figure 10.3 for an example of how to record your reps and sets for workouts 2 through 4 and for workouts 5 through 18. (See Charting Your Program Drill 3.)

Success Check

- Monitor your rest periods between sets and exercises.
- Use good exercise and spotting techniques.

Weight training workout chart (three days a week)

	Muscle area	Exercise	Training load	Set	Week — Day 1			Day 2			Day 3			Week — Day 1			Day 2		
					1	2	3	1	2	3	1	2	3	1	2	3	1	2	3
1	Chest	Bench press	90	Wt.	90			90	90		90	90		90	90		90	90	90
				Reps	13			12	12		14	12		15	14		16	15	12
2	Back	Bent-over row	80	Wt.	80			80	80		80	80		80	80		80	80	80
				Reps	12			13	12		14	13		14	14		15	14	12
3	Shoulders	Standing press	60	Wt.	60			60	60		60	60		60	60		65	65	65
				Reps	15			15	13		16	15		17	17		15	12	12
4	Biceps	Biceps curl	75	Wt.	75			75	75		75	75		75	75		75	75	75
				Reps	15			14	14		15	14		16	15		17	16	15
5	Triceps	Triceps push-down	30	Wt.	30			30	30		30	30		30	30		30	30	30
				Reps	12			12	11		14	12		15	15		17	15	13
6	Legs	Leg press	165	Wt.	165			165	165		170	170		170	170		170	170	170
				Reps	15			17	17		14	13		16	15		18	16	15
7	Abdomen	Trunk curl	—	Wt.	—														
				Reps	20			25	20		25	23		30	25		30	30	25
8				Wt.															
				Reps							2 sets						start		
9				Wt.							in workouts						3 sets		
				Reps							2, 3, 4						in workout 5		
10				Wt.													and continue		
				Reps													through		
11				Wt.													workout 18		
				Reps															
12				Wt.															
				Reps															
Body weight					140			141			140			142			141		
Date					9/23			9/25			9/27			9/30			10/2		
Comments					1 set first workout, 2 sets in workouts 2, 3, 4						3 sets starting in workout 5								

Figure 10.3 Sample record of workouts 2 through 4 followed by workouts 5 through 18.

Charting Your Program Drill 3.   *Workouts 5 Through 18*

Starting in workout 5, perform three sets of each exercise. The challenge is to keep the loads heavy or light enough so that you can perform 12 to 15 reps with excellent technique. Ask your training partner to use the technique points in steps 3 through 9 to evaluate your technique and provide feedback. Be especially concerned with breathing and controlling the speed of movement throughout the range of each exercise. Consider shortening rest periods to 45 or 30 seconds.

Record all three sets on your workout chart. Use the summary guidelines in table 10.2 to determine when and how to make changes.

Success Check

- Quality of technique is more important than the number of reps.

- Apply the two-for-two rule to keep reps between 12 and 15 in each set or between 6 and 8 reps in each set for total body exercises.

Table 10.2   Making Workout Changes Summary

Variable	Workouts 2-4	Workouts 5-18
Reps	12-15	12-15
Sets	2 sets	3 sets
Rest periods	60 sec.	30-60 sec.
Loads	Continue to make changes in loads so that they are heavy or light enough to produce 12-15 reps (except in the total body exercises).	

SUCCESS SUMMARY FOR THE STANDARD PROGRAM

In this step you learned how to transfer the exercises you selected for your program to the workout sheet in order to begin training. You also learned how to record training information on your workout sheet. Continuing to record this information in the weeks ahead is important—you will be impressed with the level of success you achieve!

Before Taking the Next Step

Honestly answer each of the following questions. If you answer yes to all of them, you are ready to move on to step 11.

1. Have you completed 18 workouts using your basic program?

2. Have you recorded your workouts on your workout chart?

3. Do you know how to modify loads so that you can complete 12 to 15 reps for each exercise and 6 to 8 reps for total body exercise (experienced)?

When you complete workout 18, which will be in six weeks if you are working out three days a week, you should begin a new training approach. To prepare, read and complete the tasks described in steps 11, 12, and 13. These steps describe how you can modify your program so that it meets your needs and interests and stimulates continued improvement.

Applying Program Design Principles

This step will help you understand the logic of designing a well-conceived weight training program. If you have trained before, the information provided here will give you a chance to determine how well your previous program followed well-accepted training principles. The elements of exercise selection, exercise arrangement, loads, reps, sets, rest-period length, and training frequency—collectively referred to as *program design variables*—are the central variables of an effective weight training program. These seven variables are grouped into the following three sections of this step:

1. Selecting and arranging exercises
2. Manipulating program variables, including training loads, number of reps, number of sets, and length of rest periods
3. Deciding training frequency

Just as certain ingredients in your favorite food must be included in proper amounts and at the correct time, so too must the sets, reps, and loads in your workouts. The workout recipe, referred to as the *program design,* is what ultimately determines the success of your weight training program (along with your commitment to training). The exciting thing about learning about program design variables is that you can then design your own program.

SELECT AND ARRANGE EXERCISES

The exercises you select will determine which muscles become stronger, more enduring, and thicker. Plus, how you arrange, or order, the exercises in your program will affect the intensity of your workouts.

Selecting Exercises

An advanced program may include as many as 15 to 20 exercises. However, a beginning or basic program (which is what you are following) need only include one exercise for each of the large muscle areas. Muscle areas of particular importance are the chest (pectoralis major), biceps (biceps brachii), triceps, shoulders (deltoids), back (latissimus dorsi, trapezius, rhomboids), hips and thighs (quadriceps, hamstrings, and gluteal muscles), and abdomen (rectus abdominis and obliques).

In steps 3 through 8, you selected one exercise for each major muscle group if you were new to weight training and one more for each area if you were experienced. Experienced trainees were also prompted in step 9 to consider including a total-body exercise. Regardless of your level of experience, you should now consider selecting more exercises for muscle areas not worked in the basic program, such as the forearm and low back; doing so will give you an even more rounded program.

If you are training to improve your athletic performance, consider adding one or both of the total-body exercises described in step 9. They involve multiple large muscle groups and explosive, power-oriented movements.

Now is also the time to consider adding exercises for muscle areas that are weak or in which you would like additional tone or size. You may also want to consider exchanging one of the basic exercises for one of the others described in each step, especially if the change means you will now perform a free-weight version of a machine-based exercise. Before making a final decision about which exercises to select, be sure you understand the exercise technique involved and the following concepts and principles.

• **Apply the specificity concept.** Your task is to identify which muscle groups you want to develop, then determine which exercises will recruit or use those muscles. This involves applying the *specificity concept*. This important concept refers to training in a manner that will produce outcomes specific to that method. For example, developing the chest requires exercises that recruit chest muscles, whereas developing the quadriceps requires exercises that recruit the quadriceps muscles.

Even the specific angle at which muscles are called into action determines if and to what extent they will be stimulated. For example, figure 11.1 illustrates how a change in body position changes the angle at which the barbell is lowered and pushed upward from the chest. The angle of the bar's path dictates whether the middle or lower portion of the chest muscles becomes more or less involved in the exercise.

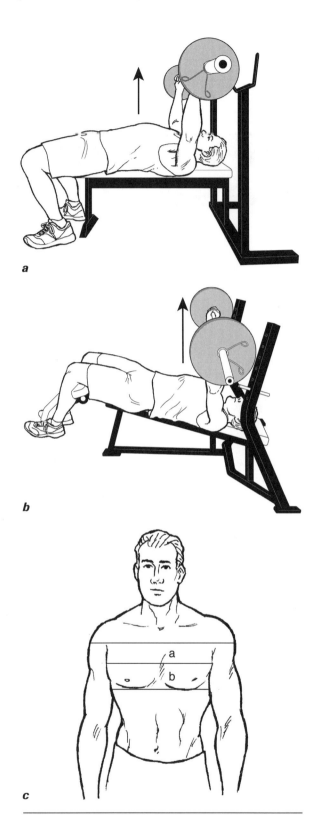

a

b

c

Figure 11.1 Effect of changing body position to alter muscle involvement. *(a)* When a horizontal position is used, the midchest becomes more involved. *(b)* When a decline position is used, the lower section of the chest becomes more involved. *(c)* These changes in body position influence muscle involvement.

The type and width of the grip are as important as body position because they too change the angle at which muscles become involved and thus the resulting effects of training. For example, using a wide grip in the bench press creates greater stress on the chest muscles than using a narrow grip does. That is why performing exercises exactly as they are described is so important.

- **Consider the need for balance.** Select pairs of exercises to help balance the strength and size of opposing muscle groups. Strength is important for creating strong joints, and size for developing a proportional physique and good posture.

Pair up opposing muscle group or body-part exercises like this:

- Chest with upper back
- Biceps with triceps
- Front (palm side) of the forearm with back (knuckle side) of the forearm
- Abdomen with the low back
- Quadriceps with hamstrings
- Front of the lower leg with the back of the lower leg

- **Consider equipment needs.** Determine the equipment needs for each exercise before making a final decision. You may not have the necessary equipment.

- **Consider the need for a spotter.** Determine whether a spotter is needed in the exercises you are considering. If one is needed but is not available, choose a different exercise to train the same muscle group.

- **Consider the time required.** Be aware that the more exercises you decide to include in your program, the longer your workouts will take. It is a common mistake to include too many! Plan for approximately 2 minutes per set unless you want a program that is designed to develop strength. If strength is your goal, you'll need to plan on about 4 minutes per set. Also, do not forget to consider the number of sets in determining the total workout time required. This is discussed in greater detail later in this step.

Arranging Exercises

There are many ways to arrange exercises in a workout. Their order affects the intensity of training and is therefore an important consideration. For instance, alternating upper- and lower-body exercises produces a lower intensity level than performing all lower-body exercises first. Exercises that involve multiple joints and muscles (multi-joint exercises) are more intense than those that involve only one joint and fewer muscles (single-joint exercises). These are the two most common arrangements:

- Perform exercises that train large muscle groups before those that train small muscles.
- Alternate exercises that involve a pushing movement with exercises that involve a pulling movement.

- **Exercise large muscle groups first (L/S).** Exercising the large (L) muscle groups before smaller (S) groups is a well-accepted approach. For example, rather than exercising the triceps (S), then the chest (L), perform the chest exercises first. Note that although the muscle area of the upper arms can appear to be large, the front and back of the arm are considered separate, small muscle groups. An example of the sequence for training large muscle groups before small muscles is shown in table 11.1.

Table 11.1 Exercise Arrangement: Large Muscle Groups First

Exercise	Type (L/S)	Muscle group
Lunge	L	Thigh and hip
Bench press	L	Chest
Lat pull-down	L	Upper back
Triceps extension	S	Back of the arm
Biceps curl	S	Front of the arm
Standing heel raise	S	Calf

• **Alternate push exercises with pull exercises (PS/PL).** You may also arrange exercises so that those that extend joints alternate with those that flex joints. Extension exercises require you to push, whereas flexion exercises require you to pull—thus the name of this arrangement, push (PS) with pull (PL). An example would be the triceps extension (PS), followed by the biceps curl (PL). This is a good arrangement because the same muscle or body area is not trained back-to-back; that is, the same muscle group is not worked two or more times in succession. This arrangement should give your muscles sufficient time to recover. An example of this method of arranging exercises is shown in table 11.2.

Table 11.2 Exercise Arrangement: Alternate Push (PS) With Pull (PL)

Exercise	Type (PS/PL)	Muscle group
Bench press	PS	Chest
Lat pull-down	PL	Back
Seated press	PS	Shoulder
Biceps curl	PL	Front of the arm
Triceps extension	PS	Back of the arm
Knee curl	PL	Back of the thigh
Knee extension	PS	Front of the thigh

Two more exercise arrangement issues need to be considered since both affect the intensity of your workout.

• **Sets performed in succession versus alternating sets.** When you are going to perform more than one set of an exercise, you will need to decide whether you will perform them one after another (in succession) or alternate them with other exercises. The following shows an example of two exercises performed for three sets in succession and alternated:

• In succession = shoulder press (set 1), shoulder press (set 2), shoulder press (set 3); biceps curl (set 1), biceps curl (set 2), biceps curl (set 3)

• Alternated = shoulder press (set 1), biceps curl (set 1), repeated until three sets of each exercise are performed

In each of these arrangements, three sets of the shoulder press and the biceps curl exercises are performed, each with a different intervening rest period and activity. Most people prefer the in-succession arrangement because it provides a greater (and more challenging) training effect.

• **Triceps and biceps exercises after other upper-body exercises.** When arranging exercises in your program, be sure that a triceps exercise is not performed before other pushing exercises such as the bench or chest press or the standing or seated shoulder press. These pushing exercises rely on assistance from elbow-extension strength from the triceps muscles. When triceps exercises precede pushing chest or shoulder exercises, they fatigue the triceps and reduce the number of reps that can be performed and the desired effect on the chest or shoulder muscles.

The same logic applies to biceps exercises. Pulling exercises that involve flexion of the elbow, such as the lat pull-down, depend on strength from the biceps muscles. Performing the biceps curl before the lat pull-down will fatigue the biceps and reduce the number of lat pull-down reps that can be performed.

Selecting and Arranging Exercises Drill 1.

Review the exercises in steps 3 through 9. In figure 11.2, demonstrate your understanding of the specificity concept by marking in the left-hand column a "C" (to mean "correct") where an exercise and the primary muscle area it develops are correctly matched and an "I" (for "incorrect") where they are not. Can you find the four that are incorrect? Answers are on page 136.

	Exercise	Primary body area developed
___	1. Back squat	Hip and thigh
___	2. Supine triceps extension	Back of upper arm
___	3. Standing press	Back
___	4. Standing heel raise	Calf
___	5. Lunge	Hip and thigh
___	6. Bent-over row	Upper back
___	7. Trunk curl	Abdomen
___	8. Shoulder shrug	Shoulders
___	9. Upright row	Back
___	10. Concentration curl	Front of upper arm
___	11. Knee curl	Back of thigh
___	12. Lat pull-down	Chest
___	13. Knee extension	Front of thigh
___	14. Hang clean	Shoulders
___	15. Back squat	Hip and thigh

Figure 11.2 Which four pairs are incorrectly matched?

Selecting and Arranging Exercises Drill 2.

Identify the one correct and two incorrectly paired exercises. Use the letter "C" to identify the correctly paired exercises. Use an "I" to identify the two pairs that are incorrect, and then correct them. Answers are on page 137.

___ 1. Concentration curl–triceps extension

___ 2. Knee extension–back squat

___ 3. Dumbbell chest fly–bent-knee sit-up

Specificity Concept Quiz

Success Check

- Apply knowledge of the muscle locations.
- Apply knowledge of exercises in steps 3 through 9.

Balanced (Paired) Exercises Quiz

Success Check

- Apply knowledge of muscle balance.
- Apply knowledge of exercises in steps 3 through 9.

Selecting and Arranging Exercises Drill 3.

Before you are able to fully understand how to arrange exercises in a workout, you need to be able to classify exercises by type. Consider the size of the muscles, the push-pull movement patterns, and the body parts involved in each of the exercises listed in figure 11.3. Fill in the missing quiz information using the letters "L" (large-muscle exercise) or "S" (small-muscle exercise), and "PS" (pushing exercise) or "PL" (pulling exercise). Answers are on page 137.

Success Check

• Apply knowledge of muscle size.

• Apply knowledge of push-pull exercise characteristics.

• Apply knowledge of exercises in steps 3 through 9.

Arranging Exercises Quiz

	Exercise	L/S	PS/PL
1.	Dumbbell chest fly	___	___
2.	Leg press	___	___
3.	Standing triceps extension	___	___
4.	Back squat	___	___
5.	Trunk curl	___	___
6.	Preacher curl	___	___
7.	Standing press	___	___
8.	Standing heel raise	___	___
9.	Upright row	___	___
10.	Knee curl	___	___

Figure 11.3 Identify the large- and small-muscle exercises and the pushing and pulling exercises.

Selecting and Arranging Exercises Answer Key

Drill 1. Specificity Concept Quiz

	Exercise	Primary body area developed
C	1. Back squat	Hip and thigh
C	2. Supine triceps extension	Back of upper arm
I	3. Standing press	Back (should be *shoulders*)
C	4. Standing heel raise	Calf
C	5. Lunge	Hip and thigh
C	6. Bent-over row	Upper back
C	7. Trunk curl	Abdomen
C	8. Shoulder shrug	Shoulders
I	9. Upright row	Back (should be *shoulders*)
C	10. Concentration curl	Front of upper arm
C	11. Knee curl	Back of thigh
I	12. Lat pull-down	Chest (should be *upper back*)
C	13. Knee extension	Front of thigh
I	14. Hang clean	Shoulders (should be *total body*)
C	15. Back squat	Hip and thigh

Drill 2. Balanced (Paired) Exercises Quiz

C 1. Concentration curl—triceps extension

I 2. Knee extension—back squat (should be *knee extension— knee curl*)

I 3. Dumbbell chest fly—bent-knee sit-up (should be *dumbbell chest fly—bent-over row or rowing exercise, seated row, or lat pull-down*)

Drill 3. Arranging Exercises Quiz

	Exercise	L/S	PS/PL
1.	Dumbbell chest fly	L	PL
2.	Leg press	L	PS
3.	Standing triceps extension	S	PS
4.	Back squat	L	PS
5.	Trunk curl	S	PL
6.	Preacher curl	S	PL
7.	Standing press	L	PS
8.	Standing heel raise	S	PS
9.	Upright row	L	PL
10.	Knee curl	L	PL

MANIPULATE PROGRAM VARIABLES

Now that you have a better understanding of exercise selection and arrangement, you need to decide on training load, reps, sets, and rest-period length. Of these, determining training loads is the most challenging.

Training Loads

Opinions differ concerning this program design variable; however, the general consensus is that decisions should be based on the specificity concept and the *overload principle*. The overload principle asserts that each workout should place a demand on the muscles that is greater than what they are used to. Training that incorporates this principle challenges the body to meet and adapt to greater-than-normal physiological stress. As it does, it establishes a new threshold that requires even greater stress to create an overload. Introducing overload in a systematic manner is sometimes referred to as *progressive overload*.

Methods for Determining Training Loads

Determining how much load to use is one of the most confusing aspects of a weight training program—and it's probably the most important one because the load determines the number of repetitions you will be able to perform and the amount of rest you need between sets and exercises. It also influences decisions concerning the number of sets and the frequency of workouts. Two approaches can be taken to determine the amount of load to use in training.

In steps 3 through 8, you used your body weight to determine initial training loads for the basic exercises. The calculations were designed to produce light loads so that you could concentrate on developing correct technique and avoid undue stress on bones and joint structures. Your goal was to calculate a load that resulted in 12 to 15 reps. This method of determining a load is referred to as a *12-15RM method* for assigning loads. The letter *R* is an abbreviation for "repetition" and the *M* stands for "maximum," meaning the maximum amount of load that you can lift with proper technique for 12 to 15 reps.

Another method is the *1RM method*—a single (1) repetition (R) maximum (M) effort. Or, said another way, it is the maximum amount of load that you can lift for one repetition in an exercise. Although not a perfect method, it is more accurate than using body weight, especially if you have good exercise technique and are conditioned to safely handle heavier loads. It is not appropriate for a beginner, however, because it requires greater skill and a level of conditioning developed only after consistently following a weight training program for six weeks or more, depending on how in shape you were when you started.

The 1RM method of determining training loads should be used only with exercises that involve more than one joint and recruit large muscle groups that can withstand heavy training loads. Exercises with these characteristics are referred to as *core exercises*. The term *core* also indicates that these exercises are training focal points (that is, the program is built around them). The core exercises included in steps 3 through 9 are:

- Bench press (free weight) and chest press (multi- or single-unit machine) from step 3

- Standing press (free weight), seated press (multi- or single-unit machine), shoulder press (cam machine), and upright row (free weight) from step 5

- Lunge (free weight), leg press (multi- or single-unit weight machine), and back squat (free weight) from step 7

- Hang clean and push press from step 9

Before attempting to predict a 1RM, be sure you have perfected your exercise technique and have at least six weeks of training under your belt.

Regardless of the load and reps assigned for core exercises, remember to keep the number of reps at 12 to 15 for all noncore exercises. A possible exception is to gradually increase the number of reps to 15 to 30 per set in the abdominal exercises performed without weights; the rationale is that since you are using a light load (your upper-body weight), it should be easier to perform a greater number of repetitions.

There are 10 procedures or steps involved in estimating or predicting the 1RM for a core exercise. To practice, work through the following example by filling in the requested information to predict a 1RM for the free-weight bench press exercise:

1. The core exercise you have selected is
   _____.

2. Warm up by performing 1 set of 10 reps with your current 12- to 15RM load. Your current 12- to 15RM load is _____ pounds.

3. Add 10 pounds (4.5 kilograms) or a weight-stack plate that is closest to that weight. Your current 12- to 15RM load + 10 pounds = _____.

4. Perform 3 reps with this load.

5. Add 10 more pounds or the next heaviest weight-stack plate. The load from procedure 3 + 10 pounds = _____.

6. Rest for 2 to 5 minutes and perform as many reps as possible with this load. Give it your best effort!

7. Using table 11.3, fill in the name of the exercise, the reps completed, and the load used.

8. Refer to table 11.4, "Prediction of 1RM." Based on the number of reps you completed, circle the rep factor number in the right-hand column of that table.

9. Record the circled rep factor in table 11.3.

10. Multiply the rep factor by the load used to obtain the predicted 1RM. Be sure to round the load off to the nearest 5 pounds (2.25 kilograms) or weight-stack plate.

Figure 11.4 illustrates an example of applying the 10 procedures for predicting the 1RM for the free-weight bench press. In this example, six reps are performed with 120 pounds. The rep factor for six reps is 1.20, which when multiplied by 120 equals 144 pounds. Rounding 144 off to the nearest 5 pounds results in a predicted 1RM of 145 pounds.

To use the 1RM to determine a training load, multiply the 1RM by a percentage. For example, if your 1RM in the standing press is 120 pounds and you decide to use a 75-percent load, the formula for figuring the training load would be 1RM × .75 or 120 × .75 = 90 pounds. This will be discussed later in this step.

Table 11.3 Developing the Chest 1RM Prediction Load

Core exercise _Bench press_

Reps completed _6_

Rep factor

Load used	from table 11.4	Predicted 1RM
_120_ x	_1.20_ =	_144_

Predicted 1RM rounded to the nearest 5 pounds/ weight-stack plate = 1RM of _145_

Table 11.4 Prediction of 1RM

Reps completed	Rep factor
1	1.00
2	1.07
3	1.10
4	1.13
5	1.16
6	1.20
7	1.23
8	1.27
9	1.32
10	1.36

Number of reps performed

Rep factor for 6 reps

Adapted, by permission, from V. Lombardi, 1989, *Beginning Weight Training: The safe and effective way.* (Dubuque, IA: William C. Brown), 201. Reproduced with permission of the McGraw-Hill Companies.

Figure 11.4 Predicting a 1RM.

1RM-Load Self-Assessment Quiz

Mark the correct choice in each of the following statements. Answers are on page 147.

1. 1RM refers to the [___ 1-repetition maximum ___ 1-minute rest minimum].
2. The [___ lunge ___ knee extension] is an example of a core exercise.
3. The procedure for predicting the 1RM includes a total of [___ 10 ___ 20] pounds that are added to your 12- to 15RM load when performing as many reps as possible.

Increasing Loads

Lifting heavier loads as soon as you are able to complete the required number of reps is important. However, changes should not be made too soon. Wait until you can complete two or more reps above the intended number in the last set of two consecutive workouts (the two-for-two rule; see step 10). When you have met the two-for-two rule, instead of referring to the load-adjustment chart (see table 2.1, page 22), simply increase loads by 2 1/2 or 5 pounds (1 or 2.25 kilograms). The load-adjustment chart was used initially to assist with large fluctuations in the number of reps performed. You will now find that fluctuations are much smaller and that using the two-for-two rule with a 2 1/2- or 5-pound increase works well, with two exceptions: For core exercises, you may need to make heavier increases. (However, underestimating is better than overestimating the increase needed.) Also, smaller load increments are appropriate for exercises that involve smaller muscles. Use 1 1/4 to 2 1/2 pound plates (0.5 to 1.0 kilograms) to make increment changes in arm (biceps, triceps), calves, and neck exercises.

Increasing Loads Self-Assessment Quiz

Mark the correct choice in each of the following statements. Answers are on page 147.

1. The two-for-two rule concerns [___ resting 2 minutes after the second set of every exercise ___ completing 2 or more reps above the goal in the last set in two consecutive workouts].

2. Load increases for the bench press and squat exercises are likely to be [___ heavier ___ lighter] than those for the biceps and triceps exercises.

Number of Repetitions

The number of reps you will be able to perform is directly related to the load you select. As the loads become heavier, the number of reps possible becomes fewer; as the loads become lighter, the number of reps possible becomes greater. Assuming that a good effort is given in each set of exercises, the primary factor that dictates the number of reps is the load selected.

Number of Reps Self-Assessment Quiz

Mark the correct choice in each of the following statements. Answers are on page 147.

1. Heavier loads are associated with a [___ greater ___ fewer] number of reps.

2. The number of reps that can be completed is primarily based on the [___ load ___ exercise] selected.

Number of Sets

Some controversy exists as to whether multiple (two or more) sets are better than single sets for developing strength, muscle size, or muscular endurance. While one-set training works exceptionally well during the early stages (10 weeks or fewer) of training, growing research supports adding more sets to the programs of well-trained individuals.

It seems reasonable to expect that the multiple-set approach to training provides a better stimulus for continued development. The rationale is that a single set of an exercise will not recruit all the fibers in a muscle and that performing additional sets will recruit more fibers. This is because muscle fibers that were involved in the first set will not be sufficiently recovered and therefore will rely on fresh fibers (not previously stimulated) for assistance, especially if succeeding sets use an increased load.

When three or more sets are performed, the likelihood of recruiting additional fibers becomes even greater. Further support for multiple sets comes from observations of the programs followed by successful competitive weightlifters, powerlifters, and bodybuilders. These competitors rely on multiple sets to achieve a high degree of development. As you will see later, your goals for training should influence the number of sets you perform.

Another consideration in determining the number of sets is the amount of time you have for training. For instance, if you choose to rest for 1 minute between exercises in your program (for a goal of muscular size), you should plan on a minimum of 2 minutes per exercise (a minimum of 60 seconds to complete the exercise, plus 60 seconds of rest). Thus your program of seven exercises, in which you perform one set of each, should take 14 minutes. If you increase the number of sets to two, and then to three, your workout time will increase to 28 and 42 minutes, respectively (assuming a 60-second rest period after each set). The actual time for rest between sets, as you will read soon, may vary from 30 seconds to 5 minutes.

Number of Sets Self-Assessment Quiz

Mark the correct choice in each of the following statements. Answers are on page 147.

1. The fewest number of sets recommended for continued development is [___ 1 ___ 2].
2. The basis for multiple-set training is that the additional sets are thought to [___ recruit ___ relax] a greater number of muscle fibers.

Length of Rest Period

The impact of the rest period between sets on the intensity of training is not usually recognized, but it should be. Longer rest periods provide time for the energizers of muscle contraction to rebuild, enabling muscles to exert greater force. If the amount of work is the same and the rest periods are shortened,

the intensity of training increases. The length of time between exercises or sets has a direct impact on the outcomes of training.

A word of caution: Moving too rapidly from one exercise or set to another often reduces the number of reps you are able to perform because of inadequate recovery time, and you may become dizzy and nauseated.

Length of the Rest Period Self-Assessment Quiz

Mark the correct choice in each of the following statements. Answers are on page 147.

1. Longer rest periods enable you to exert [___ more ___ less] force.
2. The length of the rest period has [___ an effect ___ no effect] on the outcome of training.

Application of the Specificity Concept

The earlier discussion of the specificity concept addressed only the issue of exercise selection, but this concept is broader in scope as it relates to program design. Table 11.5 shows a continuum from 100 to 65 percent of the 1RM and the number of repetitions associated with each percentage presented. For instance, selecting a load that represents 85 percent of the 1RM should yield 6 repetitions, whereas 67 percent of 1RM should yield about 12 repetitions. Knowledge of this inverse relationship is helpful when selecting loads if a specific number of repetitions is desired.

Table 11.5 Percent of 1RM– Repetition Relationship

% of 1RM	Estimated number of reps that can be performed
100	1
95	2
93	3
90	4
87	5
85	6
83	7
80	8
77	9
75	10
70	11
67	12
65	15

Adapted, by permission, from R.W. Earle and T.R. Baechle, 2004, *NSCA's Essentials of Personal Training* (Champaign, IL: Human Kinetics), 371.

Loads, reps, sets, and rest periods are manipulated using the specificity concept in designing three different programs: muscular endurance, hypertrophy, and strength. Table 11.6 illustrates a continuum in which the variables for the percentage of 1RM, number of reps and sets, and length of the rest period are presented. It reveals that muscular endurance programs (as compared to other programs) should include lighter loads (67 percent of 1RM or less), permit 12 to 20 reps, involve fewer sets (2 or 3), and have shorter rest periods (20 to 30 seconds). In contrast, programs designed to develop strength should include heavier loads (85 to 100 percent of 1RM) with fewer reps (1 to 6), more sets (3 to 5, possibly more), and longer rest periods between sets (2 to 5 minutes). Programs designed to develop hypertrophy (muscle-size increases) should utilize reps, sets, and rest periods that fall between the guidelines for developing muscle endurance and strength.

Muscular Endurance Program

The program you have been following in this book so far is designed to develop muscular endurance. You will notice some similarities between it and the program for muscular endurance in table 11.6. The loads you are using now may permit you to perform 15, but not quite 20, reps. Also, your rest periods should be close to the suggested 30 seconds if you have made an effort to shorten them. If you choose in step 13 to continue with your muscular endurance program, do not increase the load until you are able to perform 20 reps in the last set in two consecutive workouts, and keep the rest periods at 20 to 30 seconds. Except for specific situations, such as training for competitive aerobic endurance events, rest periods of less than 20 seconds are not recommended or needed.

Table 11.6 Specificity Concept Applied to Program Design Variables

Relative loading	Outcome of training	% of 1RM	Repetitions	Sets	Rest period between sets
Light	Muscular endurance	60-67	12-20	2-3	20-30 sec.
Moderate	Hypertrophy	67-85	6-12	3-6	30-90 sec.
Heavy	Muscular strength	85-100	1-6	3-5	2-5 min.

Muscular Endurance Program Self-Assessment Quiz

Write or mark the correct choices in each of the following statements. Answers are on page 147.

1. The guidelines to use when designing a program for muscular endurance are:
   a. Relative loading _____
   b. Percentage of 1RM load _____
   c. Reps _____
   d. Sets _____
2. Unless there is a specific reason, the appropriate amount of rest between sets and exercises in a muscular endurance program is [___ 10 to 15 seconds ___ 20 to 30 seconds].

Hypertrophy Program

If you decide in step 13 to emphasize hypertrophy, refer to table 11.7 to see one method of implementing the guidelines in tables 11.5 and 11.6. The example uses a 1RM of 120 pounds in the bench press exercise. To allow 10 reps per set, use 75 percent of the 1RM. This calculation equals 90 pounds (120 × .75 = 90).

Success in a hypertrophy program appears to be associated with the use of moderate loads (67 to 85 percent of 1RM), a medium number of reps (6 to 12) per set, 3 to 6 sets, and moderate rest periods (30 to 90 seconds between sets). A simple method for establishing 67- to 85-percent loads is to add 5 pounds to what you are using. Do this only with core exercises; keep the loads for other exercises the same and apply the two-for-two rule when making load adjustments.

Table 11.7 Sample Hypertrophy Program: Multiple Set–Same Load Training

Set	Goal reps	1RM × %1RM = training load
1	10	120 × .75 = 90 lbs.
2	10	120 × .75 = 90 lbs.
3	10	120 × .75 = 90 lbs.

Length of rest between sets = 30-90 sec.

1RM in the bench press = 120 lbs.

You may notice that successful bodybuilders usually perform many sets and do not rest very long between them. Thus they combine the multiple-set program described earlier in this step with the rest period and load guidelines presented in table 11.6 to promote hypertrophy.

Two unique methods implemented in hypertrophy programs are the *superset* and the *compound set*. A superset consists of two exercises that train opposing muscle groups, which are performed without rest between them; for example, one set of biceps curls followed immediately by one set of triceps extensions. A compound set is two exercises that train the same muscle group, performed consecutively without rest between them. An example is one set of barbell biceps curls followed immediately by one set of dumbbell biceps curls. The fact that these approaches deviate from the rest periods shown in table 11.6 does not mean that they are ineffective. The time frames indicated are only guidelines; program design variables can be manipulated in many ways to produce positive outcomes.

Hypertrophy Program Self-Assessment Quiz

Write or mark the correct answer in each of the following statements. Answers are on page 147.

1. The guidelines to use when designing a program for hypertrophy are:
   a. Relative loading _____
   b. Percentage of 1RM load _____
   c. Reps _____
   d. Sets _____
   e. Length of rest period _____

2. When two exercises for opposing muscle groups are performed without rest, this arrangement is referred to as a [___ superset ___ compound set].

Muscular Strength Program

Programs can be designed in many ways to produce significant strength gains. The two presented here are commonly used by successful powerlifters and weightlifters and are most appropriately applied to core exercises.

The first method is *pyramid training*. If you decide in step 13 to change your program to develop muscular strength, refer to table 11.8 to see one method of applying the guidelines presented in tables 11.5 and 11.6. The example uses a 1RM of 150 pounds in the bench press exercise. To calculate a load that will produce the goal of 6 reps in the first set, use 85 percent of the 1RM. (The second and third sets will be discussed later.) This calculation equals 125 pounds (150 × .85 = 127.5, rounded down to 125).

Another method that may get you close to 90 percent of a 1RM load is to add 15 to 20 pounds (6.75 to 9 kilograms) to what you are using currently in your core exercises. Remember to keep other exercise loads the same and

Table 11.8   Sample Muscular Strength Program: Pyramid Training

Set	Goal reps	1RM × %1RM = training load
1	6	150 × .85 = 125 lbs.*
2	4	150 × .90 = 135 lbs.
3	2	150 × .95 = 140 lbs.**

Length of rest between sets = 2-5 min.

* Rounded down from 127.5 lbs.

** Rounded down from 142.5 lbs.

1RM in the bench press = 150 lbs.

apply the two-for-two rule when making load adjustments.

Now, to incorporate the concept of progressive overload, you can use what is referred to as *light to heavy pyramid training,* in which each succeeding set becomes heavier; see the second and third sets in table 11.8, for example.

Increase the 85-percent 1RM (125 pounds) load to 90 percent of the 1RM (135 pounds) in the second set, and to 95 percent of the 1RM (140 pounds) in the third set. Sometimes you will need to round off loads to the nearest 5 pounds or closest weight-stack plate, as has been done with the loads in sets 1 and 3. Between each set, rest for 2 to 5 minutes. Use this approach with large-muscle (core) exercises, while performing 3 sets of 8 to 12 reps in other exercises. (Heavy loads tend to produce too much stress on the smaller muscles and joints.) Forcing yourself to lift progressively heavier loads from set to set provides the stimulus for dramatic strength gains. As training continues and the intensity of workouts increases, a time will come when training with very heavy loads is appropriate only on designated days. This will be discussed further in step 12.

Multiple sets–same load training is another popular approach used to develop strength. With this method you perform 3 to 5 sets of 2 to 6 reps with the same load in the core exercises and 3 sets of 8 to 12 reps in other exercises (table 11.9). The program can be made more aggressive by decreasing the goal reps, which means you must use heavier loads (table 11.5). Notice how the percentage of the 1RM is associated with the goal reps of 4, 3, and 2 at the bottom of table 11.9. You will find that completing the specified number of reps in set 1 is usually easy, set 2 is more difficult, and set 3 is very difficult, if not impossible. With continued training, sets 2 and 3 will become easier, and eventually you will need to increase the loads.

Table 11.9 Sample Muscular Strength Program: Multiple Sets–Same Load Training

Set	Goal reps	1RM × %1RM = training load
1	6	150 × .85 = 125 lbs.*
2	6	150 × .85 = 125 lbs.*
3	6	150 × .85 = 125 lbs.*

* Rounded down from 127.5 lbs.
Use 90% of 1RM for goal reps of 4.
Use 93% of 1RM for goal reps of 3.
Use 95% of 1RM for goal reps of 2.
Other exercises: 3 sets of 8-12 reps
1RM in the bench press = 150 lbs.

Muscular Strength Program Self-Assessment Quiz

Write or mark the correct answer in each of the following statements. Number 4 has two answers. Answers are on page 147.

1. The guidelines to use when designing your program for muscular strength are:
   a. Relative loading _____
   b. Percentage of 1RM load _____
   c. Reps _____
   d. Sets _____
   e. Length of rest period _____
2. Given a 1RM of 200 pounds and a goal of muscular strength development, the lightest load for a first set should be [___ 170 pounds ___ 140 pounds].
3. The use of sequentially heavier loads in each set of the pyramid training approach demonstrates the use of the [___ two-for-two rule ___ progressive overload principle].
4. The two muscular strength development programs described here have been referred to as [___ 1RM ___ pyramid ___ multiple set–same load ___ overload].
5. Heavier loads are not used with [___ smaller ___ larger] muscle groups because that method of training imposes too much stress on the involved muscle and joint structures.

Manipulating Program Variables Drill 1.

Loads, Reps, Sets, and Rest Periods

You have learned how the specificity concept and overload principle are used in determining loads and what the implications of these loads are on the number of reps and sets and on the length of the rest periods between exercises and sets. As a review, fill in the missing information in figure 11.5. Answers can be found in table 11.6, page 143.

Success Check

- Apply the specificity concept and overload principle in determining the relative loading, training outcome, percent of 1RM, reps, sets, and rest-period length.

Relative loading	Outcome of training	% of 1RM	Reps	Sets	Rest period between sets
	Muscular endurance		12-20		20-30 sec.
Moderate		67-85		3-6	
	Muscular strength		1-6		2-5 min.

Figure 11.5 Specificity concept applied to program design variables.

Manipulating Program Variables Drill 2.

Determining Load Ranges

This drill will give you experience in determining training loads, using either a predicted or actual 1RM, and in applying the knowledge you have gained about training loads. Using 85 pounds as the 1RM and the example shown for a hypertrophy program, determine the training-load ranges for a muscular strength and a muscular endurance program. Remember to round off numbers to the nearest 5 pounds or closest weight-stack plate. Write your answers in the blanks in figure 11.6. Answers are on page 147.

Success Check

- Remember percent of 1RMs for specific training outcomes.
- Round down load to nearest 5 pounds or closest weight-stack plate.

Goal	1RM		Training load (%)		Training-load range*
Hypertrophy	85	×	_67 to 85_ %	=	_55_ to _70 lbs._
Muscular strength	85	×	_____ %	=	_____ to _____
Muscular endurance	85	×	_____ %	=	_____ to _____

* Round down to the nearest 5 lbs. or weight-stack plate.

Figure 11.6 Determine training-load ranges for the sample muscular strength and muscular endurance programs.

Manipulating Program Variables Answer Key

1RM Load Self-Assessment Quiz

1. 1-repetition maximum
2. lunge
3. 20

Increasing Loads Self-Assessment Quiz

1. completing 2 or more reps in the last set for two consecutive workouts
2. heavier

Number of Reps Self-Assessment Quiz

1. fewer
2. load

Number of Sets Self-Assessment Quiz

1. 2
2. recruit

Length of the Rest Period Self-Assessment Quiz

1. more
2. an effect

Muscular Endurance Program Self-Assessment Quiz

1a. light
1b. 60 to 67 percent
1c. 12 to 20
1d. 2 or 3
2. 20 to 30 seconds

Hypertrophy Program Self-Assessment Quiz

1a. moderate
1b. 67 to 85 percent
1c. 6 to 12
1d. 3 to 6
1e. 30 to 90 seconds
2. superset

Muscular Strength Program Self-Assessment Quiz

1a. heavy
1b. 85 to 100 percent
1c. 1 to 6
1d. 3 to 5
1e. 2 to 5 minutes
2. 170 pounds
3. progressive overload principle
4. pyramid, multiple set–same load
5. smaller

Drill 2. Determining Load Ranges

Muscular strength: 85 to 100 percent; 70 to 85 pounds

Muscular endurance: 60 to 67 percent; 50 to 55 pounds

DECIDE TRAINING FREQUENCY

Training frequency is the last design variable to be covered before you will be challenged to design your own program. The question that needs to be answered is "How often should I train?" The frequency of your training, just like the application of the overload principle, is an essential element in establishing the proper intensity in successful programs.

To be effective, training must occur on a regular basis. Sporadic training short-circuits your body's ability to adapt. But rest between training days is as important as the actual training. Your body needs time to recover, to move the waste products of exercise out of the muscles and nutrients in so that muscles that are torn down from training can rebuild, thus increasing in size and strength. Rest and nutritious food intake are essential to muscle's continued growth.

Often people who are new to weight training become so excited with the changes in their strength and appearance that they start training on scheduled rest days. More is not always better, especially during the beginning stages of your program! If you are relatively new to weight training, you will need to insert rest days between training days evenly throughout the week. The result is a schedule that permits two to three workouts of the same exercises per week. As you become more accustomed to training, you can include additional exercises. Eventually, your program will include too many exercises to perform all in one workout, so you may decide to add another training day each week and redistribute (split up) the exercises across more workouts. This will make the length of each workout more reasonable and provide variety to your program.

For beginners, allowing at least 48 hours between workouts that train the same muscles is important. The result is a *three-days-a-week program.* Typically, this means training on Monday, Wednesday, and Friday; Tuesday, Thursday, and Saturday; or Sunday, Tuesday, and Thursday. In a three-days-a-week program, all exercises are performed each training day.

A *split program* is a more advanced method of training that involves performing some of the exercises two days a week (for example, Monday and Thursday) and the others on two other days (for example, Tuesday and Friday). A split program typically involves more exercises and sets and schedules the four training days as shown in table 11.10. On the left half of this table (Option A), exercises are split into upper body and lower body. Option B illustrates another common split-program option in which exercises for the chest, shoulders, and arms are performed on different days than leg and back exercises. Notice that in both options the exercises have been arranged so that pushing and pulling exercises are alternated, and triceps and biceps exercises follow upper-body pressing and pulling movements, respectively.

A split program offers several advantages. It spreads the exercises in your workout over four days instead of three, thereby usually reducing the amount of time required to complete each workout. This allows you to add more exercises and sets while keeping workout time reasonable. Because you can add more exercises, you can emphasize development in specific muscle groups, should you decide to do so. The program's disadvantage is that you must train four days a week instead of three.

Table 11.10 Four-Days-a-Week Split Training Program

Option A		Option B	
Monday and Thursday (upper body)		**Monday and Thursday (chest, shoulders, arms)**	
Exercise	**Type**	**Exercise**	**Type**
Bench press	Push	Chest press	Push
Lat pull-down	Pull	Upright row	Pull
Standing press	Push	Standing press	Push
Biceps curl	Pull	Preacher curl	Pull
Triceps extension	Push	Triceps push-down	Push
Abdominal crunch	Pull	Trunk curl	Pull
Tuesday and Friday (lower body)		**Tuesday and Friday (legs and back)**	
Exercise	**Type**	**Exercise**	**Type**
Lunge	Push	Leg press	Push
Knee curl	Pull	Knee curl	Pull
Standing heel raise	Push	Standing heel raise	Push
Knee extension	Pull	Knee extension	Pull
		Seated heel raise	Push
		Bent-over row	Pull
		Lat pull-down	Pull*

* All upper-back exercises are pulling exercises.

Frequency of Training Self-Assessment Quiz

Mark the correct choices in each of the following statements. Answers are on page 150.

1. Establishing the proper stimulus for improvement depends on using the overload principle and training [___ on a regular basis ___ in a sporadic manner].

2. Compared to a split program, the three-days-a-week program typically includes a [___ greater ___ fewer] number of exercises.

3. Compared to the three-days-a-week program, the workouts in a split program usually take [___ less ___ more] time to complete.

4. The [___split ___ three-days-a-week program] offers the best opportunity for emphasizing development in specific muscle areas.

Determining Training Frequency Answer Key

Frequency of Training Self-Assessment Quiz

1. on a regular basis
2. fewer
3. less
4. split

SUCCESS SUMMARY FOR PROGRAM DESIGN PRINCIPLES

A clear understanding of how to apply the specificity concept and the overload principle is the basis for well-conceived programs. Understanding and incorporating the guidelines for loads, reps, sets, and rest-period length in designing muscular endurance, hypertrophy, and muscular strength programs are the keys to meeting your specific needs.

When selecting exercises, keep in mind the specificity concept and the equipment and spotter requirements for each exercise. Also, include at least one exercise for each large-muscle group or body area and remember to select balanced pairs of exercises. Include additional exercises if you want to emphasize the development of certain muscle areas, but not so many that workouts take too long. Last, remember that how you arrange exercises and the order in which you perform them also has an impact on your success.

Training on a regular basis is essential to the success of your weight training program. Beginning programs typically begin with two or three workout days a week and may evolve into four-days-a-week split programs. The greater time commitment in split programs is offset by the advantages of being able to emphasize certain body parts because of the extra training time.

Your ability to recover from workout sessions is critical to your future training successes—more is not always better. Finally, muscles need to be nourished, especially after a challenging workout. Eating nutritious meals is essential for muscle repair and increases in size and strength.

Before Taking the Next Step

Honestly answer each of the following questions. If you answer yes to all of the questions, you are ready to move on to step 12.

1. Have you completed all of the self-assessment quizzes and checked your answers?
2. Do you understand how to manipulate training variables for different types of programs—hypertrophy, muscular endurance, and muscular strength?
3. Do you understand the specificity principle and how to apply it to create your program?

Step 12 provides strategies on how to modify or vary the program you have been following to avoid a plateau in your progress and keep you moving toward your weight training goals.

A common way to vary your program is to incorporate purposeful changes in training intensity.

Manipulating Program Variables to Maximize Results

This step builds on the discussion of exercise selection, arrangement, loads, reps, sets, rest periods, and training-frequency variables in step 11 and describes how these program design elements can be manipulated to maximize training outcomes.

If you perform the same number of sets and reps on the same days each week and with the same loads week after week, a plateau in strength will occur and you will not meet your goals for training. The program design variables need to be systematically varied or manipulated in order to promote continued improvements and avoid overtraining.

Although performing greater numbers of reps and sets and lifting heavier loads is necessary in order for improvement to continue, performing too many reps and sets with aggressive loads and without adequate rest periods can result in injury and extended muscle soreness and can aggravate existing joint problems. The goal, therefore, is to design programs that vary the overall intensity of training and provide the needed overload as well as rest to bring about maximum gains without injury.

Training variation involves systematically manipulating the variables of

- training frequency,
- exercise selection,
- exercise arrangement,
- number of reps per set,
- number of sets, and
- length of the rest periods between training sessions.

Programs that are designed to vary the intensity of training give special attention to the loads assigned or calculated for the core exercises (discussed in step 11). The greater muscle mass and more durable joint structures associated with larger muscle groups are better suited to withstand the rigors of weight training than smaller muscle groups. For this same reason, you may recall from step 11 that core exercises were identified as being appropriate for the heavier loads used in pyramid training as part of a muscular strength program.

Some of the common strategies used to vary the intensity of workouts are to

- lift heavy, light, and medium loads on different days of the week;
- increase loads from week to week; or
- change loads in a cyclical manner every two weeks or more.

These strategies should be applied to core exercises and programs designed to increase muscular strength and hypertrophy, which involve performing three or more sets of those core exercises. The loads used for noncore exercises should continue to allow 8 to 12 reps; they should be gradually increased using the two-for-two rule. Although the discussion here focuses on the loads used, you should realize that the number of reps and sets may be manipulated (and usually are) to vary training intensities.

WITHIN-THE-WEEK VARIATIONS

There are three primary methods of designing a program that includes changes in the loads lifted during one training week. Again, remember that any numerical or relative loading guidelines refer to changes made to core exercises only.

Three Days a Week, Same Load in Each Set

Table 12.1 shows you an example of a three-days-a-week workout program in which heavy (H), light (L), and medium (M) loads are varied within the week. The loads used in a particular day's workout do not change (thus the "same load in each set" name). The table uses abbre-

viations: "3 × 6" means "3 sets of 6 reps" and "2 × 8-12" indicates that you should perform 2 sets of 8 to 12 reps. If you completed 3 sets of 8 to 10 reps with 120 pounds, you would write it like this: "120 × 3 × 8-10."

Notice that in table 12.1 only the core exercises are associated with the letters *H, L,* or *M* designating the use of heavy (85 percent of 1RM for 6 reps), light (75 percent of 1RM for 10 reps), and medium (80 percent of 1RM for 8 reps) loads, respectively. Other noncore exercises use loads that permit 8 to 12 reps. Even though you may be able to, do *not* perform more than 10 reps on your light day or more than 8 reps on your medium day. Notice that Monday, the more intense training day, is followed by the least intense training day, which is then followed by a medium-intensity day so that your body has a chance to recover. This pattern repeats itself in all the training-program examples provided in this step.

Three-Days-a-Week Pyramid Approach

In step 11 you learned about the use of the pyramid approach, in which progressive load increases occur from one set to another until all sets for a specific exercise are completed. In table 12.2 you will recognize these progressive increases, but you should note that the loads used vary from 80 to 95 percent of 1RM on Monday (H), from 67 to 80 percent on Wednesday (L), and from 75 to 85 percent on Friday (M). The example uses a 1RM of 150 pounds (68 kilograms) and the loads are rounded down to the nearest 5-pound (2.25-kilogram) increment.

Table 12.1 Within-the-Week Training-Load Variation—Three Days a Week, Same Load Each Set

Exercise	Monday	Wednesday	Friday
Chest press*	H: 3 × 6	L: 3 × 10	M: 3 × 8
Bent-over row	2 × 8-12	2 × 8-12	2 × 8-12
Standing press*	H: 3 × 6	L: 3 × 10	M: 3 × 8
Biceps curl	2 × 8-12	2 × 8-12	2 × 8-12
Triceps extension	2 × 8-12	2 × 8-12	2 × 8-12
Back squat*	H: 3 × 6	L: 3 × 10	M: 3 × 8
Bent-knee sit-up	2 × 15-30	2 × 15-30	2 × 15-30

Heavy (H) = 85% 1RM; light (L) = 75% 1RM; medium (M) = 80% 1RM

*Core exercises

Table 12.2 Within-the-Week Training-Load Variation—Three Days a Week, Pyramid Approach

Monday—heavy (H)		Wednesday—light (L)		Friday—medium (M)	
% 1RM	Load (lbs.) × sets × reps	% 1RM	Load (lbs.) × sets × reps	% 1RM	Load (lbs.) × sets × reps
80	120 × 1 × 8	67	100 × 1 × 12	75	110 × 1 × 10
85	125 × 1 × 6	75	110 × 1 × 10	80	120 × 1 × 8
95	135 × 1 × 4	80	120 × 1 × 8	85	125 × 1 × 6

Current predicted 1RM = 150 lbs.

Four-Days-a-Week Heavy-Light Split Approach

Tables 12.3 and 12.4 show how a four-days-a-week (split) program can be organized to vary heavy and light loads within the week.

Table 12.3 shows the assignment of loads on Monday and Thursday for the chest, shoulders, and triceps. Table 12.4 shows load assignments on Tuesday and Friday for the legs, back, and biceps. Again, it is important not to perform more than 12 reps on your light day even if you are able to.

Table 12.3 Monday-Thursday Split Program—Chest, Shoulders, and Triceps

Exercise	Monday	Thursday
Bench press*	H: 4 × 6	L: 3 × 12
Dumbbell chest fly	4 × 8-12	3 × 8-12
Shoulder press*	H: 4 × 6	L: 3 × 12
Triceps extension	4 × 8-12	3 × 8-12
Abdominal crunch	2 × 15-30	2 × 15-30

Heavy (H) = 85% 1RM; light (L) = 67% 1RM

*Core exercises (3-5 sets, not including warm-up sets)

Table 12.4 Tuesday-Friday Split Program—Legs, Back, and Biceps

Exercise	Tuesday	Friday
Back squat*	H: 4 × 6	L: 3 × 12
Knee curl	4 × 8-12	3 × 8-12
Standing heel raise	4 × 8-12	3 × 8-12
Lat pull-down	4 × 8-12	3 × 8-12
Seated row	4 × 8-12	3 × 8-12
Low-pulley biceps curl	4 × 8-12	3 × 8-12

Heavy (H) = 85% 1RM; light (L) = 67% 1RM

*Core exercise (3-5 sets, not including warm-up sets)

WEEK-TO-WEEK VARIATIONS

Table 12.5 shows two ways to increase loads on a weekly basis. Option A involves simply scheduling a small percent increase each week. Option B also shows a small percentage of increase (Monday) each week, followed by the use of light and medium loads on Wednesday and Friday, respectively. Remember that the percentages shown apply only to core exercises.

Table 12.5 Within- and Between-Weeks Training-Load Variation

Option A: Same load each set, increases between weeks				Option B: Within- and between-week load variations			
Week	Monday	Wednesday	Friday	Week	Monday	Wednesday	Friday
1	80% 1RM	80% 1RM	80% 1RM	1	80% 1RM	70% 1RM	75% 1RM
2	83% 1RM	83% 1RM	83% 1RM	2	83% 1RM	73% 1RM	78% 1RM
3	86% 1RM	86% 1RM	86% 1RM	3	86% 1RM	76% 1RM	81% 1RM

CYCLICAL TRAINING VARIATIONS

The previously explained approaches provide variations in the intensity of training. If, however, you were to continue following such a program for an extended period of time, most likely either a plateau or an overtraining injury would occur. You will recall the earlier emphasis on the need for proper rest. Programs that continue to increase loads, reps, or sets without scheduling rest time will not produce optimal gains. The term *periodization* refers to the scheduling of cycles of high-intensity and low-intensity training periods.

A typical periodization strategy divides a program into time periods. The largest division is a *macrocycle,* which usually lasts an entire training year but may range from one month to four years (for Olympic athletes, for example). Within the macrocycle are two or more *mesocycles* that last several weeks to several months. Each mesocycle is divided into two or more *microcycles,* each of which is usually one week long.

Table 12.6 represents an eight-week cycle that includes load variations within the week for core exercises *only,* and load and set increases after every three weeks of training. Follow the guidelines for loading and sets for each heavy, light, and medium training day. On Friday of the third and sixth weeks, complete the following procedures to determine a new predicted 1RM to use when calculating the new training loads:

Table 12.6 Eight-Week Training Cycle

Week	Sets	Monday	Wednesday	Friday
1	3	H	L	M
2	3	H	L	M
3	3	M	L	Testing
4*	4	H	L	M
5	4	H	L	M
6	4	M	L	Testing
7*	4	H	L	M
8	2	L	L	L
9	Retest 1RM and repeat 8-week cycle with new training loads			

Heavy (H) = 85% 1RM; light (L) = 67% 1RM; medium (M) = 75% 1RM

* Begin using loads based on new predicted 1RM from previous Friday's testing.

1. Warm up as usual, then use Friday's loads in sets 1 and 2 (and 3 for week 6), but perform only 5 and 3 reps (6, 4, and 2 reps for week 6), respectively.

2. If you are using the pyramid method, perform as many reps as possible with the heaviest load used thus far in this cycle (specific to the exercise being tested). If you are using the same load in each set, increase the load lifted in

the last set by 10 pounds (4.5 kilograms) and perform as many reps as possible.

3. Predict the 1RM using the procedures you learned in step 11 (see page 139). A second shortcut method for identifying training loads is described in the next section.

In the fourth and seventh weeks, the loads lifted are based on new calculations using the newly tested 1RMs established during the Friday workout of the third and sixth weeks. Notice that the eighth week involves lighter loads and fewer sets (less intensive workouts), providing an opportunity for the body to recover as well as to increase strength levels in succeeding weeks. The number of sets may also be increased after each three-week period. A four-days-a-week program could be cycled in a similar way.

SHORTCUT FOR DETERMINING TRAINING LOADS

Instead of multiplying the predicted 1RM by the desired training percentage to determine training loads as you did in step 11, refer to table 12.7 and follow these steps:

1. Locate and circle your predicted 1RM value in the "1RM" column.

2. Identify the desired training percentage (50 to 95 percent).

3. Follow the percentage column down until it meets the row for your predicted 1RM value and circle that number, which is your training load.

Figure 12.1 shows an example of this shortcut. In the example, the lifter completed seven reps with 90 pounds and wants a training load that represents 85 percent of 1RM. Completing seven reps with 90 pounds equals a 1RM of 110 pounds using the procedures to predict the 1RM explained in step 11 (see page 139). In table 12.7, under the column heading "1RM," 110 pounds is found on line 9. The number at the intersection of line 9 and the 85-percent column is the calculated training load (94), which is rounded to the nearest 5 pounds or weight-stack plate (95 pounds).

Regardless of the method you use to create variations in intensity, you should perform as many reps of the core exercises as possible on the heavy days of your workout schedule, but keep them within the designated ranges during the Wednesday (light) and Friday (medium) workouts. This means that even though you may be capable of performing more reps with the lighter Wednesday and Friday loads, don't do it! In the noncore exercises, use the two-for-two rule for increasing loads.

Table 12.7 Training-Load Determination

Line	1RM	Training-load percentage							
		50%	60%	70%	75%	80%	85%	90%	95%
1	30	15	18	21	23	24	26	27	29
2	40	20	24	28	30	32	34	36	38
3	50	25	30	35	38	40	43	45	48
4	60	30	36	42	45	48	51	54	57
5	70	35	42	49	52	56	60	63	67
6	80	40	48	56	60	64	68	72	76
7	90	45	54	63	68	72	77	81	86
8	100	50	60	70	75	80	85	90	95
9	110	55	66	77	83	88	94	99	105
10	120	60	72	84	90	96	102	108	114
11	130	65	78	91	98	104	111	117	124
12	140	70	84	98	105	112	119	126	133
13	150	75	90	105	113	120	128	135	143
14	160	80	96	112	120	128	136	144	152
15	170	85	102	119	128	136	145	153	162
16	180	90	108	126	135	144	153	162	171
17	190	95	114	133	143	152	162	171	181
18	200	100	120	140	150	160	170	180	190
19	210	105	126	147	158	168	179	189	200
20	220	110	132	154	165	176	187	198	209
21	230	115	138	161	173	184	196	207	219
22	240	120	144	168	180	192	204	216	228
23	250	125	150	175	188	200	213	225	238
24	260	130	156	182	195	208	221	234	247
25	270	135	162	189	203	216	230	243	257
26	280	140	168	196	210	224	238	252	266
27	290	145	174	203	218	232	247	261	276
28	300	150	180	210	225	240	255	270	285
29	310	155	186	217	233	248	264	279	295
30	320	160	192	224	240	256	272	288	304
31	330	165	198	231	248	264	281	297	314
32	340	170	204	238	255	272	289	306	323
33	350	175	210	245	263	280	298	315	333
34	360	180	216	252	270	288	306	324	342
35	370	185	222	259	278	296	315	333	352
36	380	190	228	266	285	304	323	342	361
37	390	195	234	273	293	312	332	351	371
38	400	200	240	280	300	320	340	360	380

Table 11.4   Prediction of 1RM

Reps completed	Rep factor
1	1.00
2	1.07
3	1.10
4	1.13
5	1.16
6	1.20
8	1.27
9	1.32
10	1.36

⑦ reps = ──→ ⟨1.23⟩ ──────→ × 90 = ⟨110 lbs.⟩ (rounded)

Adapted, by permission, from V. Lombardi, 1989, *Beginning Weight Training: The safe and effective way.* (Dubuque, IA: William C. Brown), 201. Reproduced with permission of the McGraw-Hill Companies.

94 rounded to the nearest 5 lbs. = 95-lb. training load

Table 12.7   Training-Load Determination

Line	1RM	Training-load percentage					
		50%	60%	70%	75%	80%	85%
1	30	15	18	21	23	24	26
2	40	20	24	28	30	32	34
3	50	25	30	35	38	40	43
4	60	30	36	42	45	48	51
5	70	35	42	49	52	56	60
6	80	40	48	56	60	64	68
7	90	45	54	63	68	72	77
8	100	50	60	70	75	80	85
9	110	55	66	77	83	88	94
10	120	60	72	84	90	96	102
11	130	65	78	91	98	104	111
12	140	70	84	98	105	112	119
13	150	75	90	105	113	120	128
14	160	80	96	112	120	128	136
15	170	85	102	119	128	136	14'
16	180	90	108	126	135	144	1'

Figure 12.1   A shortcut for determining training loads.

Program Variation Self-Assessment Quiz

Mark the correct choice in each of the following statements. Answers are on page 159.

1. The reps performed on light and medium training days allow you to [___ apply the overload principle ___ recover from the overloading].

2. You should perform [___ the designated number of reps ___ as many reps as possible] on heavy training days.

3. The two variables that have been manipulated in the eight-week training cycle in table 12.6 are [___ reps and sets ___ loads and sets].

Maximizing Training Drill 1. *Shortcut Method*

This drill is designed to give you experience in the shortcut method of determining training loads using table 12.7. Assume that you performed the "as many reps as possible test" with 150 pounds and were able to complete 8 reps. If you want to use 75 percent of 1RM, what is the correct training load? Remember to use the procedures for predicting the 1RM (see table 11.4, page 139) from step 11 first, and then use this 1RM value and the 75 percent 1RM column of table 12.7 to locate the correct training load. Round off this value to the nearest 5-pound increment or weight-stack plate. The answer is on page 159.

Success Check

- Associate the number of reps completed with the rep factor (see table 11.4).
- Multiply the rep factor by the load lifted to determine the predicted 1RM.
- Locate and circle where your predicted 1RM value is located in the "1RM" column (see table 12.7).
- Identify the desired training percentage column.
- Identify the intersecting point to determine the training load.

Maximizing Training Drill 2. *Determining Training Loads in a Program*

To give you another opportunity to determine training loads, fill in training loads for the program shown in figure 12.2. In this drill, assume that 5 reps were performed with 105 pounds. Answers are on page 159.

Success Check

- Associate the number of reps completed with the rep factor (see table 11.4, page 139).

- Multiply the rep factor by the load lifted to determine the predicted 1RM.
- Locate and circle the predicted 1RM value on table 12.7.
- Multiply the desired training percentage by the predicted 1RM.
- Round off loads.

	Monday (H)	Wednesday (L)	Friday (M)
Week 1	80% 1RM = _____	67% 1RM = _____	75% 1RM = _____

Figure 12.2 Practice determining training loads. Assume 5 reps were performed with 105 pounds.

Answer Key

Program Variation Self-Assessment Quiz

1. recover from the overloading

2. as many reps as possible

3. loads and sets

Maximizing Training Drill 1.   Shortcut Method

The load that should be lifted to perform as many reps as possible is 150 pounds. Using table 11.4, we find that the rep factor for 8 reps is 1.27. We multiply 150 pounds by 1.27 to get 190.5 pounds. On table 12.7, 190 pounds is on line 17. Line 17 intersects with the 75-percent column at 143. Rounded off, this number equals a training load of 145 pounds.

Maximizing Training Drill 2.   Determining Training Loads in a Program

The load used is 105, with gives us a rep factor of 1.16 for 5 reps, according to table 11.4. If we multiply 105 by 1.16, we get 121.8 pounds, which rounds to 120 pounds as the predicted 1RM. We find 120 pounds on line 10 in table 12.7. For a training load of 80 percent, find the number at the junction of line 10 and 80 percent in table 12.7 (96, rounded down to 95). For a training load of 67 percent, we would multiply 120 by .67 for a result of 80.4 pounds (rounded to 80). For a training load of 75 percent, find the number at the junction of line 10 and 75 percent in table 12.7 (90 pounds).

Monday: 80 percent of 1RM = 95 pounds

Wednesday: 67 percent of 1RM = 80 pounds

Friday: 75 percent of 1RM = 90 pounds

SUCCESS SUMMARY FOR PROGRAM VARIABLES

Training intensity can be varied in many ways, but the most common methods involve manipulating the amount of the load, the number of sets and reps, and the number of training days. The use of periodization programs that include aggressive training weeks followed by a week (or weeks) of less aggressive training provide an appropriate overload and an opportunity for the body to recover and make significant gains.

As you become more experienced, you may want to learn more about periodization. Detailed discussions can be found in the texts by Earle and Baechle (2004), Baechle and Earle (2000), Fleck and Kraemer (2003), and Lombardi (1989).

Before Taking the Next Step

Honestly answer each of the following questions. If you answer yes to all of the questions, you are ready to move on to step 13.

1. Have you completed the self-assessment quiz and the drills and checked your answers?
2. Do you understand how to manipulate training variables to maximize training?
3. Can you calculate new training loads using table 11.4 and table 12.7?

Step 13, the last step, allows you to apply everything you have learned about developing your own weight training program. You will be prompted to use your knowledge about the program-design variables described in the last two steps and apply the overload and specificity concepts to design a program that meets your needs. Enjoy the challenge!

Creating Your Program

This is your chance to apply all that you have learned to create your own weight training program. In this step, you will use your knowledge of program design variables and apply the overload and specificity concepts to design a program that meets your needs. If you follow the procedures in this step as they are presented, you will develop a well-conceived, individualized weight training program. You may also use these tasks to assess your level of comprehension about how to design a weight training program.

Follow this order when developing your program:

1. Determine your training goal.
2. Select exercises.
3. Decide on training frequency.
4. Arrange exercises.
5. Calculate your training loads.
6. Decide how many reps to perform.
7. Decide how many sets of each exercise to complete.
8. Decide on the length of rest periods.
9. Decide how to vary the program.

DETERMINE YOUR TRAINING GOAL

Think about why you want to weight train and which results or outcomes you desire. Place a check mark next to your most important training goal, then read the paragraphs that follow to understand which type of program will allow you to meet your goal.

My most important training goal is to improve my (*choose one*)

Muscular endurance

Hypertrophy

Muscular strength

General muscular toning

Body composition (reproportioning)

Other (describe: _____

_____)

Choosing a single training goal will help you focus your efforts and maximize your results, but it does not prevent you from selecting a new primary training goal when you are ready to make a change!

• **Goal—muscular endurance.** As you have learned, your present program is designed to improve muscular endurance. If this is the outcome you want from training, you will not need to make many changes. Simply try to increase the number of reps from 15 to 20 in the core exercises and increase the numbers of sets for all exercises. If possible, also try to reduce the length of the rest periods between sets and exercises.

• **Goal—hypertrophy.** To produce hypertrophy, you need to use loads that will keep your reps between 8 and 12, and you probably will need to include a higher number of exercises and sets. You may want to initially focus on chest and arm development, but avoid the common tendency to spend so much time on those body parts that you exclude or minimize workouts to develop your legs. Also be aware that as you increase the number of exercises, sets (to as many as 6), and days of training, the amount of time you will need to commit to your program will increase substantially.

• **Goal—muscular strength.** If muscular strength is your goal, you will need to handle loads that are quite a bit heavier than you are currently using. An important thing to remember (from step 11) is that to safely and effectively handle the heavier loads associated with developing strength, you must have fairly long rest periods (2 to 5 minutes) between sets. A common mistake is to rush through sets. Doing so slows recovery and compromises your ability to exert a maximum effort in succeeding sets. Additionally, remember that only your core exercises can be assigned heavy loads (85 percent of 1RM or heavier) and lifting those loads will require several warm-up sets and a spotter.

• **Goal—general muscle toning.** Follow the guidelines presented for muscular endurance programs to meet this goal. If you do not experience satisfactory changes in muscle tone from that type of program, switch to a program designed to produce hypertrophy.

• **Goal—body composition (reproportioning).** If reproportioning your body is your goal, it is likely that you believe you are carrying too much body fat, not enough muscle, or both. Consider doing three things: Follow a hypertrophy training program to increase muscle mass, select your foods more carefully, and begin an aerobic exercise program to increase the number of calories you expend. For the hypertrophy program, simply follow the guidelines presented in this text. When selecting foods, make sure that you eat a balanced diet, increase your intake of complex carbohydrates, and decrease your intake of fats. Most normal diets will supply the needed amount of protein. For more information on nutrition, refer to the book by Clark (2003). For directions on how to design an aerobic exercise program, use the texts by Baechle and Earle (2005) or Hoeger (1995).

• **Goal—other.** If you have special needs, such as improving athletic performance in weightlifting, powerlifting, or other sports activities, read the chapter by Baechle and Conroy (1996), and texts by Baechle and Earle (2000), Earle and Baechle (2004), Fleck and Kraemer (2003), Garhammer (1986), and Komi (2002) and journals published by the National Strength and Conditioning Association. You'll find helpful guidelines for designing and implementing programs for young athletes in the text by Faigenbaum and Westcott (2000). If your interest is bodybuilding, consult the text by Sprague (1996). The texts by Westcott and Baechle (1997 and 1999) will be helpful for those interested in programs designed specifically for older populations, and the book by Baechle and Earle (2005) is helpful if you are looking for sample programs for body shaping, muscle toning, strength, or cross-training.

SELECT EXERCISES

The exercises included in your current program are few, but they work most of the major muscle areas of the body. It is a basic program that will benefit from the addition of exercises for the low back, forearm, and other small muscle areas.

If your goal is to increase muscular endurance, muscle size, or muscular strength in a particular body part, adding another exercise that is designed to train those muscles is a good idea. If you add exercises, do not select more than two per muscle area at this time, and do not include more than a total of 12 exercises if you are following a three-days-a-week program. As you will remember from step 11, the four-days-a-week split program allows you to add more exercises. Thus you may choose to include three exercises for a particular body part if you decide to follow a four-days-a-week program.

Using table 13.1, decide which of the muscle areas listed you want to select exercises for or to which you want to add emphasis (meaning you already have one exercise for this muscle area and you want to add one more). Before

Table 13.1 Exercise Selection

Days	Muscle area	Exercises
	Total body	
	Chest	
	Back (upper)	
	Shoulders	
	Triceps	
	Biceps	
	Hip/thigh	
	Calves	
	Abdomen	

completing this task, you may want to refer to steps 3 through 9 to review the explanations and descriptions of the various free-weight and machine exercises. Remember to consider the equipment needed and the spotter requirements. After considering your goals, write the name of the exercise to the right of the appropriate muscle areas.

DECIDE ON TRAINING FREQUENCY

Decide whether you are going to use a three-days-a-week or four-days-a-week (split) program. If you decide on a split program, determine how you will divide the exercises among the four days. You may need to reconsider the number of exercises you have selected. Remember, you can include more exercises in split programs than in a three-days-a-week program.

Choose how often you plan to weight train:

- Three days a week (If you chose this option, skip to the next section on arranging exercises.)

- Four-days-a-week split program (If you chose this option, go down to the next line.)

For a split program, choose which schedule you will follow:

- Chest, shoulders, and triceps on two days; legs, back, and biceps on the other two days

- Upper body on two days; lower body on the other two days

Once you make these decisions, go back to table 13.1 and, under the "Days" column, write which days of the week you plan to perform each exercise.

ARRANGE EXERCISES

Next decide how you will arrange these exercises within a workout. Step 11 pointed out several options. Choose which arrangement you plan to use:

- Exercise large muscle groups first.
- Alternate push exercises with pull exercises.

Now look again at the exercises that you want to include in your program and decide how you will determine the order in which you will perform them. Rewrite the names of the exercises, in order, on table 13.2 using the left-hand column if you plan to follow a three-days-a-week program and the right-hand column for a four-day (split) program.

Table 13.2 Exercise Arrangement

Three-days-a-week program		Four-days-a-week split program	
Order	**Exercise**	**Order**	**Exercise**
1		Monday/Thursday exercises	
2		1	
3		2	
4		3	
5		4	
6		5	
7		6	
8		7	
9		Tuesday/Friday exercises	
10		8	
11		9	
12		10	
		11	
		12	
		13	
		14	

Now record the exercises in the proper order from table 13.2 on the chart in figure 13.1 (for a three-days-a-week program) or figure 13.2 (for a four-days-a-week program). The four-days-a-week chart assumes that you are training Monday/Thursday and Tuesday/Friday.

Weight training workout chart (three days a week)

Name _____

Muscle area	Exercise	Load × sets × reps	Set	Week ___ Day 1					Day 2					Day 3				
				1	2	3	4	5	1	2	3	4	5	1	2	3	4	5
1			Wt.															
			Reps															
2			Wt.															
			Reps															
3			Wt.															
			Reps															
4			Wt.															
			Reps															
5			Wt.															
			Reps															
6			Wt.															
			Reps															
7			Wt.															
			Reps															
8			Wt.															
			Reps															
9			Wt.															
			Reps															
10			Wt.															
			Reps															
11			Wt.															
			Reps															
12			Wt.															
			Reps															

Body weight _____

Date _____

Comments _____

From *Weight Training: Steps to Success, Third Edition*, by Thomas R. Baechle and Roger W. Earle, 2006, Champaign, IL: Human Kinetics.

Figure 13.1 Workout chart for a three-days-a-week program.

Weight training workout chart (four days a week)

Name _____

Monday/ Thursday exercises	Load × sets × reps	Set	Week																					
			Day 1–Monday					Day 2–Tuesday					Day 3–Thursday					Day 4–Friday				
			1	2	3	4	5	1	2	3	4	5	1	2	3	4	5	1	2	3	4	5
1		Wt.																					
		Reps																					
2		Wt.																					
		Reps																					
3		Wt.																					
		Reps																					
4		Wt.																					
		Reps																					
5		Wt.																					
		Reps																					
6		Wt.																					
		Reps																					
7		Wt.																					
		Reps																					

Tuesday/Friday exercises	Load × sets × reps	Set	Day 1–Monday					Day 2–Tuesday					Day 3–Thursday					Day 4–Friday				
			1	2	3	4	5	1	2	3	4	5	1	2	3	4	5	1	2	3	4	5
8		Wt.																				
		Reps																				
9		Wt.																				
		Reps																				
10		Wt.																				
		Reps																				
11		Wt.																				
		Reps																				
12		Wt.																				
		Reps																				
13		Wt.																				
		Reps																				
14		Wt.																				
		Reps																				
Body weight																						
Date																						
Comments																						

From *Weight Training: Steps to Success, Third Edition,* by Thomas R. Baechle and Roger W. Earle, 2006, Champaign, IL: Human Kinetics.

Figure 13.2 Workout chart for a four-days-a-week program.

CALCULATE YOUR TRAINING LOADS

Based on the overload principle, the specificity concept, your primary training goal, and the type of exercise (core or noncore), determine the warm-up and workout load for each exercise.

First select your approach. Review the explanations of the different approaches presented in step 11. Decide which approach you will take when deciding on the amount of load to use for each exercise:

12-15RM method

1RM method

You may want to use both methods, especially if you are well trained and will begin a program that gives higher intensities to core exercises. If so, you should make a list of which exercises will be assigned loads from which approach.

If you are following a muscular strength program, you need to identify the approach you will follow:

Pyramid training

Multiple sets–same load training

Now determine starting loads. Using the guidelines presented in step 11 for core and noncore exercises, calculate the loads for the exercises selected. To save time, you can use the shortcut method of determining training loads from step 12. Record these loads on the chart in figure 13.1 (three days a week) or figure 13.2 (four days a week split) in the "Load × sets × reps" box. Leave room for the sets and reps numbers. Do this now, but take your time because this process is the most important of all of the program design variables.

DECIDE HOW MANY REPS TO PERFORM

Based on your primary training goal, the load calculations from the previous task, and table 11.6 (see page 143), determine the number of reps you intend to perform in each set:

12 to 20 reps

6 to 12 reps

1 to 6 reps for core exercises and 8 to 12 reps for noncore exercises

Other (describe: _____

_____)

Fill in the number of reps for each exercise in the "Load × sets × reps" box next to the loads you just wrote in. Leave room for the number of sets.

DECIDE HOW MANY SETS OF EACH EXERCISE TO COMPLETE

Depending on how well trained you are, what your training goal is, and how much time you have to work out, decide on the number of sets you plan to perform for each exercise listed on

your workout chart in the "Load × sets × reps" box. You might want to assign more sets to the core exercises.

DECIDE ON THE LENGTH OF REST PERIODS

Based on your training goal, decide how much rest you will allow yourself between sets and exercises:

20 to 30 seconds (for muscular endurance)

30 to 90 seconds (for hypertrophy or the noncore exercises of a muscular strength program)

2 to 5 minutes (for muscular strength)

You may also want to allow yourself a little extra time between sets of a new exercise so that you do not become too fatigued and perform it incorrectly.

DECIDE HOW TO VARY THE PROGRAM

Consult step 12, if necessary, and then decide which method you will use to vary load intensities:

Within-the-week variation (heavy, light, medium days)

Between weeks or week-to-week variation

Cyclical variation (periodization)

If you chose the within-the-week variation, decide which approach you will take to vary the loads lifted in the core exercises:

Same load in each set

Pyramid

Heavy–light split

If you chose the between-weeks variation, decide which approach you will take to vary the loads lifted in the core exercises:

Same load in each set with increases between weeks

Within- and between-week load variations

If you chose the cyclical variation, decide when you will make load increases for the core exercises:

Weekly

Every two weeks

Other (describe: _____
_____)

Now decide how you plan to make load increases for the core exercises:

Increase loads by a specified percentage. (How much? ___ percent)

Increase loads based on retesting. (How often to retest? Every ___ weeks)

Finally, decide on the number of training weeks that you will complete before a week of low-intensity training is scheduled:

4 weeks

5 weeks

6 weeks

7 weeks

8 weeks

Program Design Drill. *Design an Eight-Week Program*

Depending on which method of program variation you plan to follow, fill in the loads, reps, and sets for all exercises for a eight-week period on a separate sheet of paper.

Success Check

- Select one primary training goal.
- Select exercises.
- Decide on training frequency.
- Arrange exercises.
- Calculate training loads.
- Determine number of reps to perform.
- Determine number of sets of each exercise to complete.
- Decide on the length of the rest periods.
- Decide how to vary the program.

SUCCESS SUMMARY FOR CREATING YOUR PROGRAM

The activities included in this step required you to apply everything you have learned about how to design a weight training program. You are capable of designing a program that meets your current needs, but you may want to look ahead and consider how to modify or manipulate the program design variables during the next year.

In the process of learning about equipment, exercise techniques, and program design variables, you have probably gained a better appreciation of the expertise required to design programs for athletes in various sports and programs for special populations (prepubescents, seniors, pregnant women, and those with osteoporosis, hypertension, or injuries). If you fall into one of these categories, or if you are training such individuals, you may want to refer to the texts by Baechle and Earle (2000), Earle and Baechle (2004), and Fleck and Kraemer (2003).

Remember, no program will allow you to reach your training goal unless you approach it with a positive attitude. If you train hard, train smart, and eat sensibly, you are guaranteed success and the opportunity to enjoy wearing your workouts proudly.

◨ Glossary

absolute strength—A comparative expression of strength based on actual load lifted.

adipose tissue—Fat tissue.

aerobic—In the presence of oxygen.

aerobic capacity—A measurement of physical fitness based on maximum oxygen uptake.

aerobic energy system—The metabolic pathway that requires oxygen for the production of adenosine triphosphate (ATP).

aerobic exercise—Exercise during which the muscle cells receive enough oxygen to continue at a steady state. Some examples are walking, biking, running, swimming, and cross-country skiing.

all-or-none law—A muscle cell that is stimulated by the brain will contract maximally or not at all; a stimulus of insufficient intensity will not elicit a contraction.

alternated grip—A grip in which one hand is supinated and the other hand is pronated, so that both thumbs point in the same direction. Also called a mixed grip, it is used for spotting the bench press (see step 3).

amino acids—Nitrogen-containing compounds that form the building blocks of protein.

anabolic—Tissue building that is conducive to the constructive process of metabolism.

anabolic steroid—Testosterone, or a substance resembling it, which stimulates body growth anabolically as well as androgenically.

anaerobic—In the absence of oxygen.

anaerobic exercise—Exercise during which the energy needed is provided without the utilization of inspired oxygen. Examples include weightlifting and the 100-meter sprint.

androgen—Any compound that has masculinizing properties.

assistance exercises—Exercises that supplement the core exercises. For example, the knee extension exercise may be used as a supplement to the squat, a core exercise.

atrophy—A decrease in the cross-sectional size of a muscle fiber due to lack of use, disease, or starvation.

barbell—A piece of free-weight equipment that is used in two-arm exercises; a long bar on which weight plates may be placed on both ends.

basal metabolic rate (BMR)—The amount of energy, expressed in kilocalories, that the body requires to carry on its normal functions at rest.

bodybuilding—A sport that involves weight training to develop muscle hypertrophy. Bodybuilders are judged on their muscle size, definition, symmetry, and posing skill.

body composition—The quantification of the body's components, especially fat and muscle. It can be measured by various methods, such as skin-fold calipers, girth measurement, impedance, and underwater (hydrostatic) weighing.

calorie—The measure of the amount of energy released from food or expended in metabolism (exercise). The standard unit, a kilocalorie (Kcal or calorie), is 1,000 calories but is usually incorrectly termed a "calorie."

carbohydrate (CHO)—A group of chemical compounds composed of carbon, hydrogen, and oxygen. Examples include sugars, starches, and cellulose. It is a basic foodstuff that contains approximately 4 kilocalories per gram.

cardiac muscle—A type of striated (involuntary) muscle tissue located only in the heart.

cardiorespiratory fitness—This category of fitness ("cardio" refers to the heart, "respiratory" to the lungs) pertains to the efficiency of the heart and lungs in delivering oxygen to the working muscles.

circuit training—A variation of interval training that uses weights and timed work and rest periods. This type of weight training program is typically designed to increase muscular endurance.

closed grip—A grip in which the fingers and the thumbs are wrapped (closed) around the bar.

collar—The part of a barbell or dumbbell that keeps weight plates from sliding toward the hands.

common grip—A grip in which the hands are placed at roughly shoulder-width, equidistant from the weight plates.

compound set—Two exercises that work the same muscle group, which are performed consecutively without resting between them. For example, a compound set for the chest would be a set of the bench press followed immediately by a set of the dumbbell chest fly. Often misnamed a "superset."

concentric muscular action—A type of muscular action characterized by tension being developed followed by the muscle shortening (e.g., the upward phase of a biceps curl).

conditioning—A process of improving the capacity of the body to produce energy and do work.

cool-down—The period in which an individual performs light or mild exercise immediately after completing a training session. Its primary purpose is to facilitate the movement of blood back to the heart and enable the body to gradually return to a resting state.

core exercises—The primary weight training exercises that stress the large muscle groups of the body.

cycles—A specific period of time (weeks, months, or years) over which the frequency, volume, and intensity of training are systematically varied to avoid overtraining and to promote continued progress.

cycling—Systematically changing the frequency, volume, and intensity of training.

dumbbell—A piece of weight training equipment, typically used in single-arm exercises, that consists of a short bar with weight plates on each end.

dynamic—Exercise involving movement; its opposite is *static*.

dynamic muscle action—Involves movement and consists of concentric, eccentric, or both types of muscle activity.

eccentric muscular action—A muscular action in which there is tension in the muscle; however, the muscle lengthens rather than shortens. An example can be seen in the lowering phase of the biceps curl, where the biceps muscles are lengthening even though there is tension in the muscle. Eccentric muscle actions are associated with the muscle soreness commonly experienced in weight training.

ergogenic aid—A substance used to enhance performance.

essential fat—The fat stored in the bone marrow as well as in the heart, lungs, liver, spleen, kidneys, muscles, and lipid-rich tissues throughout the central nervous system. A minimum value of 3 percent for males and 12 percent in females is required for normal physiological functioning.

exercise prescription—An exercise program based on present fitness levels and desired goals or outcomes.

extension—A movement occurring at a joint that increases its angle. The downward movement of the triceps push-down is an example of elbow extension.

fast-twitch fiber—A type of skeletal muscle fiber that is highly recruited during explosive muscular activities such as sprinting, shot putting, and competitive weightlifting.

fat—Essentially nonmetabolically active tissue that contains approximately 9 kilocalories per gram and should constitute 25 to 30 percent of the diet.

fixed-resistance machine—A weight training machine in which the location of the weight stack does not move, resulting in an inconsistent load during exercise.

flexibility—The ability of a joint to move through its available range of motion.

flexion—A movement occurring at a joint that decreases its angle. The upward movement of the biceps curl is an example of elbow flexion.

free weight—An object such as a barbell or dumbbell that is used for physical conditioning and competitive lifting.

frequency—The number of training sessions in a given time period; for example, three times a week.

handoff—An assist by the spotter in moving a bar off its supports for the lifter.

hormone—A chemical substance secreted by an endocrine gland that has a specific effect on activities of other cells, tissues, and organs.

hydrostatic weighing—A method of body-composition determination that utilizes underwater weighing and calculation of body volume and density. Generally accepted as one of the most accurate methods of determining body composition.

hyperplasia—An increase in muscle size due to muscle fibers splitting and forming separate fibers.

hypertension—High blood pressure.

hypertrophy—An increase in the cross-sectional area of the muscle. More simply stated, an increase in muscle size.

hyperventilation—Excessive ventilation of the lungs due to increased depth and frequency of breathing, usually resulting in the elimination of carbon dioxide. Accompanying symptoms include low blood pressure, dizziness, and rapid breathing.

intensity—The relative stress level that an exercise stimulus places on the appropriate system.

ischemia—A condition in which the supply of oxygen to working tissues is reduced.

isokinetic—A type of muscular activity in which contractions occur at a constant velocity as controlled by an ergometer. The term describes only a concentric muscle action.

isometric (or static) contraction—A type of muscular activity in which there is tension in the muscle, but it does not shorten. Either the bony attachments are fixed or the forces that would lengthen the muscle are countered by forces that are equal to or greater than those generated by the muscle to shorten.

isotonic—Implies a dynamic event in which the muscle generates the same amount of force through the entire movement. Such a condition occurs infrequently, if at all, in human performance; therefore, the word should not be employed to describe human exercise performance. In loose terms, however, it is used to describe dynamic free-weight exercises and some machine exercises.

kilocalorie (Kcal)—A unit of work or energy equal to the amount of heat required to raise the temperature of 1 kilogram of water 1 degree Celsius. A quantity of energy equal to 1,000 calories.

lean body weight—Body weight minus fat weight; nonfat or fat-free weight.

ligament—Dense connective tissue that attaches the articulating surfaces of bones together.

load—The amount of weight lifted for a repetition.

locks—On barbells or dumbbells, mechanisms that are located on the outside of the weight plates, which hold the plates on the bar.

macrocycle—A time period or cycle of training within a periodized training program that typically lasts from one month to one year.

mesocycle—A time period within a periodized training program that typically lasts several weeks to a month; two or more mesocycles are part of a macrocycle.

metabolism—The sum total of the chemical changes or reactions occurring in the body.

microcycle—A time period or cycle of training within a periodized training program that is part of a mesocycle and typically lasts one to four weeks.

motor unit—An individual motor nerve and all the muscle fibers it innervates (stimulates).

movement pattern—The line of travel of the body and the bar or equipment during a repetition.

multiple sets—Performing more than one set of an exercise (after a rest period) before moving to a different exercise.

muscle-bound—A term that has been used to describe people who weight train as having limited joint flexibility, which can be due to a lack of muscle activity or to chronic use of poor lifting and stretching methods. The term is inappropriate to describe those who practice sound weight training techniques and proper stretching exercises.

muscular endurance—The capacity of a muscle to repeatedly contract over a period of time without undue fatigue. This is a local muscle characteristic.

muscular strength—The capacity of a muscle to exert maximally one time. This is a local muscle characteristic often expressed as 1RM.

Nautilus—A brand of dynamic resistance training equipment.

negative exercise—A form of exercise, more appropriately termed *eccentric exercise,* in which the muscle lengthens rather than shortens.

neuromuscular—Involving both the nervous and the muscular systems.

nutrition—The study of food and how the body uses it. The sum total of the processes involved in taking in food and the subsequent metabolic effects.

Olympic bar—A bar approximately 7 feet long that has rotating sleeves on the ends to hold the weights. The diameter of the bar is about 1 inch in the middle and 2 inches at the ends. It weighs 45 pounds; with Olympic locks, typically 55 pounds.

Olympic weightlifting—A form of competitive lifting that involves a contest of maximum strength levels in the clean and jerk and the snatch.

one-repetition maximum (1RM)—The resistance (load) with which an individual can perform only 1 repetition using a maximum effort.

open grip—A hand position, sometimes referred to as a false grip, in which the thumbs are not wrapped around the bar.

overhand grip—The hands grip a bar so that the palms are pronated (face down) or away.

overload principle—Progressively increasing the intensity or volume of workouts over the course of a training program as exercise tolerance improves.

overtraining—A state of undue mental or physical fatigue (or both) brought about by excessive training without sufficient rest.

oxygen uptake—The ability of the heart and lungs to take in and utilize oxygen. Commonly expressed in milliliters of oxygen per kilogram of body weight per minute (ml/kg/min).

percent body fat—The percentage of body weight that is comprised of fat, or the ratio of fat to fat-free weight. Recommended ranges are 14 to 18 percent for men and 22 to 26 percent for women.

periodization—A method of varying a training program that schedules cycles of high-intensity and low-intensity training periods.

physical fitness—A product of a high level of cardiorespiratory endurance, muscular strength, muscular endurance, and flexibility combined with a low ratio of body fat to lean body weight.

powerlifting—A competitive sport that involves contesting strength levels in the back squat, bench press, and deadlift exercises.

progressive resistance—Gradually increasing a load (intensity) over time to bring about desired improvements.

pronated grip—Grasping a bar at midbody height so that the palms face down and the thumbs face each other. Also termed an overhand grip.

prone—Lying face downward; the opposite of supine.

progressive overload—Introducing overloads in a systematic manner.

protein—A food substance, containing approximately 4 kilocalories per gram, that provides the amino acids essential for tissue growth and repair.

pyramid training—A method of multiset training in which loads get progressively heavier or lighter.

quick-lift exercise—A weight training exercise characterized by explosive movements; examples include the power clean, snatch, and hang clean.

range of motion (ROM)—The available movement through which a body part rotates about a joint.

recruitment—The activation of motor units by the neuromuscular system during muscular activity.

relative strength—A comparative measure of strength based on a variable, such as total body weight or lean body weight.

repetition—The execution of an exercise one time.

repetition maximum (RM)—The maximum load that a muscle group can lift over a given number of repetitions before fatiguing. For example, a 10RM load is the maximum that can be lifted for 10 repetitions.

resistance training—Any method or form of exercise that requires a person to exert force against resistance.

rest interval—A given amount of time between sets or exercises.

set—In weight training, the number of repetitions consecutively performed in an exercise without resting.

skeletal muscle—A type of muscle tissue that attaches to bone via tendons and responds to voluntary stimulation from the brain.

slow-twitch fiber—A type of skeletal muscle fiber that has the ability to repeatedly work without undue fatigue. This type of muscle fiber is highly recruited for long-distance running, swimming, and cycling events.

smooth muscle—A type of involuntary muscle tissue located in the eyes and in the walls of the stomach, intestines, bladder, uterus, and blood vessels.

specificity of training—The idea that one should train in a specific manner for a specific outcome.

split system (split routine)—A weight training program characterized by scheduling certain exercises (for example, upper-body or lower-body exercises) on alternate days.

squat rack—Supports (sometimes called *standards*) that hold a barbell at shoulder height; typically used in placing the bar on a lifter's back for the squat exercise.

standard bar—A bar used for weight training that is 1 inch (2.5 centimeters) in diameter and typically weighs approximately 5 pounds (2.25 kilograms) per foot.

static stretch—Involves holding a static position, passively placing the muscles and connective tissues on stretch.

sticking point—The point in the range of motion of an exercise at which moving the weight or resistance is most difficult.

strength plateau—A temporary leveling off of progress in a strength training program.

strength training—The use of resistance training to increase one's ability to exert or resist force for the purpose of improving performance. The training may utilize free weights, a person's own body weight, machines, or other devices to attain this goal.

striated muscle—Skeletal muscle that possesses alternate light and dark bands, or striations. Except for the cardiac muscle, all striated muscles are voluntary.

superset—A set in which two exercises that train opposing muscle groups are performed without rest between them.

supinated grip—Grasping a bar held at mid-body height so that the palms face upward and thumbs point in opposite directions. Also termed an underhand grip.

supine—Lying on the back, facing upward; the opposite of prone.

supplemental exercise—Exercises used in addition to core exercises to intensify the training of a certain muscle or muscle group. Sometimes referred to as assistance or noncore exercises.

tendon—Dense connective tissue that attaches a muscle to a bone.

testosterone—A hormone responsible for male sex characteristics.

underhand grip—The hands grip a bar held at midbody height so that the palms face upward (supinated) while the thumbs face away from each other.

underwater weighing—A technique utilized to determine body density. Knowing the density of the body, the percentage of body fat can be calculated. Also termed hydrostatic weighing.

Universal—A brand of dynamic resistance equipment.

variable-resistance machine—A weight machine in which the location of the weight stack varies to create a more consistent load during exercises.

variation—Manipulating the frequency, intensity, duration, or mode of an exercise program to promote maximal improvements with minimal opportunities for overtraining, either mentally or physically.

vitamin—An organic material that acts as a catalyst for vital chemical (metabolic) reactions.

volume—The total workload per exercise, session, or week. In weight training, the volume is proportional to the total number of repetitions times the total amount of weight. Sometimes volume is defined as sets times the number of reps.

warm-up—A period in which an individual performs light or mild exercise immediately before a training session. Its primary purpose is to prepare the body for more intense exercise.

weight training—Exercises performed using free weights, machines, or other forms of resistance for the purpose of increasing strength, muscular endurance, or muscle size.

◪ References

Baechle, T. R., and B. P. Conroy. 1996. Preseason strength training. In *Team physician's handbook.* 2nd ed. Ed. M. Mellion, M. Walsh, and G. Shelton. New York: Hanley and Belfus.

Baechle, T. R., and R. W. Earle. 2000. *Essentials of strength and conditioning.* 2nd ed. National Strength and Conditioning Association. Champaign, IL: Human Kinetics.

Baechle, T. R., and R.W. Earle. 2005. *Fitness weight training.* 2nd ed. Champaign, IL: Human Kinetics.

Baechle, T. R., and B. R. Groves. 1994. *Weight training instruction: Steps to success.* Champaign, IL: Human Kinetics.

Baechle, T. R., and B. R. Groves. 1994. *Weight training steps to success video.* Champaign, IL: Human Kinetics.

Clark, N. 2003. *Nancy Clark's sports nutrition guidebook.* 3rd ed. Champaign, IL: Human Kinetics.

Corbin, C., and R. Lindsey. 1997. *Concepts of physical fitness with laboratories.* 9th ed. Dubuque, IA: W.C. Brown.

Earle, R. W., and T. R. Baechle. 2004. *NSCA's essentials of personal training.* Champaign, IL: Human Kinetics.

Faigenbaum, A., and W. Westcott. 2000. *Strength and power for young athletes.* Champaign, IL: Human Kinetics.

Fleck, S. J., and W. J. Kraemer. 2003. *Designing resistance training programs.* 3rd ed. Champaign, IL: Human Kinetics.

Garhammer, J. 1986. *Sports Illustrated strength training.* New York: Harper & Row.

Hoeger, W. K. 1995. *Lifetime fitness, physical fitness, and wellness.* 4th ed. Englewood, CO: Morton.

Komi, P. V. 2002. *Strength and power in sport (Encyclopedia of sports medicine series).* Champaign, IL: Human Kinetics.

Kraemer, W. J., and T. R. Baechle. 1989. Development of a strength training program. In *Sports medicine.* 2nd ed. Ed. J. Ryan and F. L. Allman Jr. San Diego, CA: Academic Press.

Lombardi, V. P. 1989. *Beginning weight training: The safe and effective way.* Dubuque, IA: W. C. Brown.

Sprague, K. 1996. *More muscle.* Champaign, IL: Human Kinetics.

Stone, M. H. 1993. Position statement on anabolic-androgenic steroid use by athletes. National Strength and Conditioning Association. Colorado Springs, CO: NSCA.

Westcott, W. L. 2003. *Building strength and stamina.* 2nd ed. Champaign, IL: Human Kinetics.

Westcott, W. L., and T. R. Baechle. 1997. *Strength training past 50.* Champaign, IL: Human Kinetics.

Westcott, W. L., and T. R. Baechle. 1999. *Strength training for seniors.* Champaign, IL: Human Kinetics.

◱ About the Authors

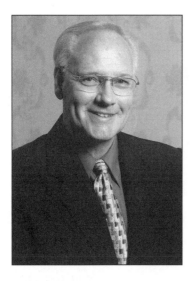

Thomas R. Baechle, EdD, CSCS,*D; NSCA-CPT,*D, a former competitor in Olympic-style weightlifting and powerlifting, was a weight training instructor and a strength and conditioning coach for 20 years. He also directed a phase III cardiac rehabilitation program for 16 years. Currently he holds the rank of professor and is chair of the exercise science and athletic training department at Creighton University. He is a cofounder and past president of the National Strength and Conditioning Association (NSCA) and executive director of the NSCA Certification Commission. Baechle has been recognized as the force behind the creation of the Certified Strength and Conditioning Specialist and NSCA-Certified Personal Trainer examination programs. He has received the NSCA's two most coveted awards: Strength and Conditioning Professional of the Year and Lifetime Achievement. He has served as president of the National Organization of Competency Assurance and on various regional, national, and international boards. Dr. Baechle has authored, coauthored, or edited 12 books, 2 of which have been translated into 10 languages, including the popular *Fitness Weight Training,* coauthored by Roger Earle.

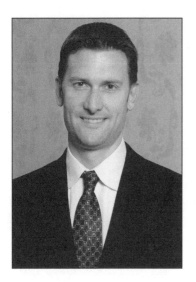

Roger Earle, MA, CSCS,*D; NSCA-CPT,*D, is associate executive director and director of examination development for the NSCA Certification Commission. He is responsible for reviewing and editing the CSCS and NSCA-CPT exams and developing study resources with Thomas Baechle, including *Essentials of Strength Training and Conditioning* and *NSCA's Essentials of Personal Training.*

Earle's 20 years of experience as a personal trainer, combined with his roles as a college weight training instructor and a Division I strength and conditioning coach, prepared him well for his numerous national and international conference presentations on the topic of designing strength training programs for athletes of all sports and fitness levels. Earle received his undergraduate and master's degrees in exercise science. At Creighton University, he was a Division I strength coach for nine years and a faculty member of the exercise science and athletic training department for eight years.

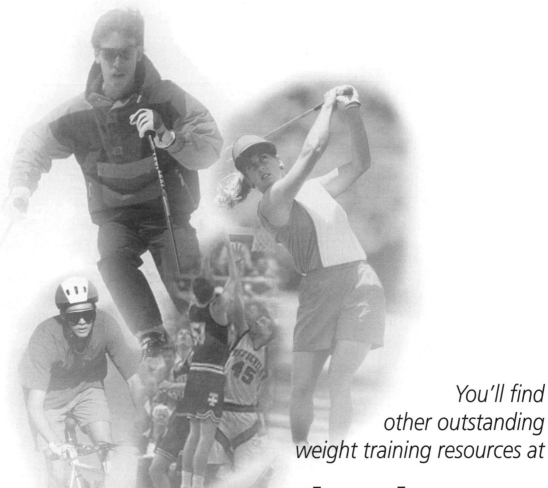